CHILD REARING

INFLUENCE ON PROSOCIAL AND MORAL DEVELOPMENT

J.M.A.M. JANSSENS
J.R.M. GERRIS
(EDITORS)

INSTITUTE OF FAMILY STUDIES,
UNIVERSITY OF NIJMEGEN, THE NETHERLANDS

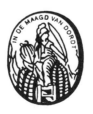

SWETS & ZEITLINGER B.V. AMSTERDAM / LISSE

PUBLISHING SERVICE

Library of Congress Cataloging-in-Publication Data

[applied for]

Cip-gegevens Koninklijke Bibliotheek, Den Haag

Child

Child rearing: influence on prosocial and moral development / ed. J.M.A.M. Janssens, J.R.M. Gerris. - Amsterdam [etc.] : Swets en Zeitlinger
Met lit. opg.
ISBN 90-265-1181-7
NUGI 721
Trefw.: opvoeding / ontwikkelingspsychologie.

Typesetting: Athmer/SKP, Utrecht
Cover design: Rob Molthoff
Cover printed by Casparie, IJsselstein
Printed in the Netherlands by Offsetdrukkerij Kanters B.V., Alblasserdam

ISBN 90 265 1181 7
NUGI 721

Contents

J.M.A.M. Janssens & J.R.M. Gerris

Introduction

This book examines relations between child rearing and children's prosocial and moral development. The four chapters of Part I deal with relations between child rearing and children's prosocial development, and the four chapters of Part II with relations between child rearing and their moral development. In each part, the first two chapters describe review studies and the last two empirical studies.

In Chapter 1, Holden and Coleman discuss the advantages and disadvantages of interviews, questionnaires, and observations to assess child-rearing behavior. They review 16 studies on relations between child rearing and the prosocial development of children. Most studies rely on questionnaires and interviews; only two utilized observational data. Holden and Coleman thus conclude that research on relations between child rearing and children's prosocial development is characterized by an over-reliance on self-report data. Moreover, they found an over-emphasis on parental reactive behavior; in most studies, child-rearing behavior is operationalized as child discipline. Parental discipline responses are only a part of child rearing. Nonreactive parental behavior (modeling, affection, teaching) also influences the child's development. However, it received less attention than disciplinary techniques in these studies. Holden and Coleman provide three suggestions to assess child rearing more accurately and comprehensively. First, we should sharpen our conception of parental behavior. A clearer conceptualization of parenting would account for parental actions as well as reactions. Second, we should develop a new self-report device that is less susceptible to interview-related bias, but is more flexible and interactive than the reflective questionnaire methodology. Third, we need more advanced multivariate statistical methods to reveal the nature and consequences of parent-child relations.

In most studies, prosocial development is operationalized as prosocial behavior. Prosocial behavior means action on behalf of someone else involving a net cost to the actor. Examples of prosocial behavior are sharing, comforting or helping someone in distress, or making a donation to someone in need. Another aspect of prosocial development concerns prosocial moral reasoning, i.e. reasoning about conflicts where the individual has to choose between satisfying his or her own wants or needs and those of others in contexts where laws, punishments, authorities, formal obligations, and other external criteria are irrelevant or deemphasized. The development of prosocial moral reasoning in childhood and midadolescence is the main theme of Chapter 2. Based on cross-sectional and longitudinal studies, Eisenberg and Miller delineated an age-related development sequence of prosocial moral reasoning. Stages in this sequence include hedonistic reasoning, need-oriented reasoning, empathic reasoning, and reasoning from internalized norms. The stage of a child's reasoning in a situation depends on several factors (e.g. situational factors, personality, own values and, values of others). One of these factors is socialization. In the research described by Eisenberg and Miller, differences in reasoning are found between American children and children from Germany, Israel and Papua New Guinea. The differences reflect different cultural values. From research on socialization of prosocial development, Eisenberg and Miller also conclude that children's level of prosocial moral reasoning is related to parental support, nonrestrictiveness, and parental emphasis on autonomy and responsibility. Thus socialization may not only influence prosocial behavior, as is demonstrated by Holden and Coleman in the first chapter, but research is also presented showing that reasoning about prosocial issues is influenced by child-rearing behavior.

In Chapter 3, both of the aspects of prosocial development, the behavior and the reasoning, are examined. Janssens and Gerris found positive relations between prosocial reasoning and several indices of prosocial behavior. Moreover, they noted that both aspects of prosocial development are dependent on child-rearing behavior. In their study, child-rearing behavior is assessed by interviewing children about their parents. Janssens and Gerris did not confine their study to the influence of child discipline (induction and power assertion), but also looked for relations between prosocial development and other parental behavior components such as support and demandingness. They noted that different child-rearing behavior components are not independent of each other. Demandingness, induction, and support are positively related to each other and negatively to power assertion. All the child-rearing behavior components examined in this study appear to be related to children's prosocial development. Perceived parental support, demandingness, and induction are positively related to prosocial development, and power assertion is negatively related to prosocial development. Janssens and Gerris also studied the mediating function of empathy between child rearing and the child's prosocial development. They noted that empathy has a positive effect on prosocial development, and that the child's empathy is infuenced by a child-rearing style characterized by induction and demandingness. These results indicate a mediating role of empathy between child rearing and prosocial development. However, the relation between child rearing and prosocial development is not exclusively mediated by empathy. First, the relations between empathy and child rearing, and between empathy and prosocial development are weak. Second, Janssens and Gerris noted a direct effect of support on prosocial development; other factors than empathy thus still play a role in mediating and explaining the relations between child rearing and prosocial development.

In Chapter 4, Iannotti et al. report on a longitudinal study of child rearing, empathy, and prosocial behavior. Mothers and children were observed when the children were two and five years old. The mothers also completed a questionnaire about child-rearing attitudes. Iannotti et al. noted increased prosocial behavior at the age of five. However, there were no significant correlations between the children's prosocial behavior at two and at five. As far as child rearing is concerned, Iannotti and his colleagues noted a positive relation between maternal attitudes and behavior and they found that the mothers' child-rearing patterns exhibited some extent of stability. Moreover, it seems that a child's prosocial behavior is influenced by several parental behavior components: maternal warmth, nurturance, expression of affect, and rational direction of the child's behavior. Like Janssens and Gerris, Iannotti and his colleagues also looked for mediating links between child rearing and prosocial behavior. They found, however, little reason to suggest a mediating link of socio-cognitive processes (e.g. empathy, perspective taking) between child rearing and the children's prosocial behavior.

The second part of the book focuses on relations between child rearing and moral development. In Chapter 5, Power and Manire study relations between child rearing and moral internalization. Moral internalization means that the concern for others is displayed independently of the fear of punishment or the hope of reward by external agents. According to Power and Manire, for internalization to occur, children have to develop (1) an understanding of the appropriateness, desirability, or acceptability of a given act, (2) the ability to regulate their behavior in response to societal demands, and (3) an internal motivation to comply to these demands. Parents can encourage the development of internalized behavior in their children by (a) establishing a warm and supportive relationship with their child, (b) communicating clear expectations for appropriate behaving, (c) using only minimal significant external pressure to ensure compliance, and (d) providing the social information children need to make responsible, independent decisions. These relations between child rearing and moral internalization are presented in the second part of Power and Manire's chapter. In the first part, they study the socialization goals parents have, and developmental trends in these goals. Parents of toddlers stress household rules, parents of pre-schoolers focus on encouraging responsible interpersonal behavior, parents of children in middle childhood encourage assertiveness and initiative, and parents of adolescents focus on independence. These shifts in goals are reflected in shifts in child-rearing behavior. As children grow older, parents provide them with increasing opportunities for self-regulation. They make their children more and more responsible for their own behavior.

In most studies, a distinction is drawn between internalization and compliance. In the case of compliance, children are motivated by their expectations for external rewards and punishments; in the case of internalization, the motivation is internal. According to Kuczynski (Chapter 6), this is an undifferentiated conception of compliance. Kuczynski distinguishes between three categories of compliance: externally motivated compliance, internally motivated compliance, and receptive compliance. Externally motivated compliance is primarily motivated by incentives based on parental use of force or parental control over material resources. Internally motivated compliance is primarily maintained by motivational resources within the child. Inductive parental strategies are necessary for internally motivated compliance, whereas power assertion is effective to elicit immediate externally motivated compliance. Receptive compliance is a form of compliance that stems from a generalized willingness on the part of children to cooperate with their parents. This willingness is positively related to secure attachment and to parental responsiveness. The conception of non-compliance is usually undifferentiated. It is mainly viewed as undesirable. In the last part of his chapter, Kuczynski argues that some level of non-compliance is a positive sign of children's developing autonomy. It is important that parents are able to discriminate among different forms of non-compliance, and to provide differential feedback to the child for appropriate and inappropriate forms of non-compliance.

In Chapter 7, De Veer and Janssens report on a study of relations between victim-oriented child rearing, perspective taking, and moral internalization. According to De Veer and Janssens, several types of induction can be distinguished which may have different effects on child development. They hypothesize that messages directing the child's attention toward the victim are particularly likely to stimulate moral internalization, since they directly appeal to the the child's perspective-taking ability. De Veer and Janssens studied two aspects of moral internalization: guilt and moral behavior. They noted that perspective taking is positively influenced by victim-oriented discipline and that perspective taking has a positive effect on guilt and moral behavior. These findings support the hypothesis that perspective taking mediates between victim-oriented discipline and moral internalization. Victim-oriented discipline, however, also directly influences guilt. This influence is not mediated by the child's capacity to take perspective. At any rate, De Veer and Janssens did not find any relation between guilt and moral behavior. Feelings of guilt are thus not sufficient conditions for moral behavior.

In Chapter 8, Janssen, Janssens, and Gerris studied another aspect of moral development, moral reasoning. Moral reasoning refers to the arguments used to justify a moral judgment. Kohlberg distinguished six stages of moral reasoning. Based on increasing complexity, these six stages can be placed in a developmental order. Each successive stage exhibits an increased moral-cognitive competence. Janssen, Janssens, and Gerris noted that parents who reason about moral issues at higer stages more frequently use inductive discipline techniques than parents who reason at lower stages. They also noted that induction is positively related to a child's stage of moral reasoning. From these two results, it can be concluded that the relation between parental moral reasoning and a child's moral reasoning is mediated by child discipline. In a Lisrel-analysis, Janssen, Janssens, and Gerris found evidence of an indirect influence of maternal and paternal moral reasoning on the child's moral reasoning. Moreover, they noted also a direct influence of maternal moral reasoning on the child's moral reasoning. There have to be other mediating processes to explain the relation between parental moral reasoning and the child's stage of moral reasoning.

Based on the results and conclusions from the eight studies reported in this book, there are three central issues future child-rearing research should focus upon. First, very little is known about the relationship between indices of prosocial and moral development. In this book, prosocial behavior, prosocial reasoning, moral behavior, moral internalization, and moral reasoning are examined, but hardly anything is known about the relations between these concepts. Second, regarding the influence of child-rearing behavior on prosocial and moral development, there is consistent evidence of a positive influence of child-rearing behavior components such as support, affection, responsiveness, inductive child discipline, encouragement of independence and responsibility. However, correlations between child-rearing measures and indices of prosocial and moral behavior are rather low. Several authors argue that these low correlations are due to poor conceptualizations and measurements of parental behavior. If their objections are valid, we have to look for alternative conceptions and measures of child rearing. Third, very little is known about the factors and processes that play a mediating role between child rearing and prosocial and moral development. In some studies, empathy and perspective taking are studied as mediating links between child rearing and children's prosocial and moral development, but there is very little evidence of these mediating relations.

G.W. Holden & S.D. Coleman

The Measurement of Child Rearing: Paradox and Promise

The task of measuring parental behavior has been a goal of psychology since the recognition of the fundamental and unique role parents play in children's development. Ostensibly, measuring how parents rear their children is a relatively simple and straight-forward task. Because we all have some familiarity with child rearing, there is no shortage of subjects, and the phenomenon is readily visible, the measurement of parenting should not be hard. In contrast to expensive and esoteric instruments such as magnetic resonance imaging used by neurologists to measure neurological structures, or partical accelerators used by physicists to identify sub-atomic particles, the measurement of child rearing is within the grasp, technical expertise, and expense account of almost any interested scientist. For all these reasons, the measurement of child rearing appears to be a relatively easy task.

In actuality, we will argue that the measurement of child rearing is deceptively *difficult*. The difficulty of the task, in the face of the apparent ease creates a paradox. It is unfortunate that the difficulty of this task has gone largely ignored; the failure to appreciate the paradox has been a major obstacle in developing better conceptualizations of child rearing and methods for measuring parental behavior, and been at the expense of scientific progress. That is not to say the accurate measurement of child rearing cannot be attained; however, there is much work to be done before that can be achieved.

This chapter will be organized around revealing the difficulties inherent in measuring child rearing, with illustrations from the research on child rearing and prosocial development. To begin, the three basic methods that have been used to measure child rearing will be reviewed and briefly evaluated. A prototypic study using each method will be briefly described. Next we will examine the success with which researchers have measured child rearing in conjunction with prosocial development. To do that we will first summarize the ways in which parents have been thought to facilitate—or impede—children's prosocial development. Then a methodological review of the literature that has linked parenting with children's prosocial behavior will follow. That will be followed by a more general discussion of common methodological pitfalls associated with the measurement of child rearing. The chapter will end with suggestions for future work in order to more fully and accurately measure child rearing.

Basic Methods

Currently, three methods are used commonly by researchers to measure child rearing: questionnaires, interviews, and observations.

Questionnaires. Questionnaires or surveys are the oldest and most popular tool for the measurement of child rearing; their origins can be traced back to the beginning of psychology in this country (Sears, 1899). Since the 1930s they have been utilized widely. Given their prevalence, it follows that child-rearing surveys represent a heterogeneous group of instruments; they differ in terms of their structure and length, the content, and who serves as respondents.

The one standard feature of any questionnaire is, of course, that it is presented and answered on paper. After that, the variation begins. Items on the questionnaires have appeared in the form of rating adjectives on a semantic differential scale, responding to phrases or single sentences using Likert-type ratings, selecting a multiple choice response following a short vignette, or having to remember items from a list of items. *By far, the most common format utilized has been the Likert-type scale, where phrases are responded to on an agree-disagree rating scale.* The number of items on the questionnaires has also varied considerably—from less than 10 items to over 400!

The content of the surveys have been directed at a variety of child-rearing topics and domains of parental social cognition. The great majority of child-rearing questionnaires are designed purportedly to assess global child-rearing attitudes. Upon closer inspection of the surveys, it is clear that they do not only assess parental attitudes (or predisposition, reaction to, or affective evaluation of the supposed facts), but many include questions assessing a variety of domains in parents' social cognition. The most common domains include the more general values (abstract goals or a coherent set of attitudes), specific beliefs (ideas that could be disproved), self perceptions (reactions or feelings about parenting or children), and behavioral intentions (orientations toward behavioral practices). Some of the newer parent questionnaires have avoided this potpourri of items and constructed surveys that measure only one domain, such as beliefs (e.g., Roehling & Robin, 1986) or behavioral intentions (e.g., Crase, Clark, & Pease, 1979).

When questionnaire items do, in fact, probe parental global attitudes, such as warmth or control, they are typically assessed with decontextualized statements (e.g., "A good mother loves her child"). It has been commonly assumed that generalized attitudes provide a convenient and short-cut way to document parental behavior and reveal individual differences between parents. Holden and Edwards (1989), in an exhaustive review, identified 83 instruments designed to measure parents' attitudes published through 1986. Well over 100 different global child-rearing attitudes concerning parents' views on family matters, parent-child interactions, and children's social and cognitive development have been assessed.

To date, the single most frequently used child-rearing survey has been the Parent Attitude Research Instrument (PARI), developed by Earl Schaefer and Richard Bell (1958). The PARI is a 115-item survey that is responded to on a 4-point Likert-type agree-disagree scale. The survey contains 23 five-item subscales, including marital conflict (e.g., "Sometimes it's necessary for a wife to tell off her husband in order to get her rights"), strictness with child ("A child will be grateful later on for strict training"), and acceleration of development ("The sooner a child learns that a wasted minute is lost forever the better off he will be"). Results from the subscales are assumed to reflect stable attitudes; these attitudes are presumed to influence or even determine parental behavior.

Both parents and their children have been called upon to fill out child-rearing questionnaires. Mothers have been the most common respondent, but more recently fathers have been included. In some cases, both parents have independently filled out surveys in order to assess the concordance of child-rearing views (e.g. Block, Block, & Morrison, 1981). The recipients of the child rearing, the children themselves, have also filled out surveys about their parents since

Stogdill piloted the approach in 1937. In fact, enough studies had collected children's reports of their parents' behavior to warrant a review over 20 years ago (Goldin, 1969). This topic continues to be actively investigated with a number of different questionnaries, with the presupposition that it is the child's subjective perception of parental behavior, rather than the child-rearing behavior itself, that may have the most important impact on the child.

Interviews. The second major tool for assessing child rearing is the parental interview. Hoffman (1957) championed the use of interviews as a way to obtain data about behavior that is otherwise difficult to observe or the act of observing could interfere with the activity being observed. It was also regarded as affording an efficient substitute for observations, and allowing probes and flexibility in questionning, something not possible with paper and pencil surveys. As a result, greater detail and precision about child-rearing practices and attitudes could be measured.

The format of interviews, like questionnaires, has varied widely. Most interview schedules adopt an approach somewhere in the middle of the extremes of flexible, unstandardized dialogues, to highly structured interview where the respondent verbally selects one response from a list of multiple choice questions. The number of questions asked has ranged from fewer than 20 to 185 questions.

The classic and prototypic interview study of child rearing was published in the same year that Hoffman advocated the use of interviews. Robert Sears and his colleagues, published their influential study of the effects of child rearing based on the interview data from 379 mothers of 5-year-old children (Sears, Maccoby, & Levine, 1957). Their partially open-ended interview schedule consisted of about 72 main questions with follow-up questions for a total of 185 questions. Questions included current and retrospective maternal attitudes and practices ("How often do you spank your child"; "How about when he was younger—say two or three years old"), maternal reports of paternal attitudes and practices ("How does your husband feel about strict obedience"), and reports of child behavior ("How much attention does your child seem to want from you"). From those two hours of tape-recorded interviews, transcriptions were made, and then 188 rating scales were created.

Interviews for measuring child rearing continue to appear periodically in the literature, but much less frequently than questionnaires. For example, of the 154 instruments developed since 1974 to measure characteristics of parenthood, 83% were questionnaires and only 9% were interviews (Holden, 1990). The remaining 8% were observational instruments, the third basic tool for measuring child rearing.

Observations. Observations are fundamentally different from questionnaires and interviews because they do not rely on self-report data. A second difference is that the method measures overt child-rearing practices, the ultimate focus of the other two types of instruments. Observations can be divided into two major types: observations reduced into ratings and observations reduced into behavioral units. Ratings involve the summary judgments of an observer, who after watching the parent, makes a series of ratings of the parent's behavior. Or behavior can be observed and measured by some type of behavioral unit—such as the number of times some event occurred. This latter type has been labelled "systematic observations" (Bakeman & Gottman, 1986).

The first extensive effort to collect observations of parents was conducted by Alfred Baldwin and his colleagues in 1945 (Baldwin, Kalhoun, & Breese, 1945). Parents and their 4-year-old children, who were serving as participants in a longitudinal study conducted by the Fels Research Institute, were observed periodically in their homes. Observers then rated each parent on 30 bipolar ratings scales (e.g., dictatorial vs. democratic, withholds help vs. over-helps, hostile vs. affectionate) that had been developed by Champney (1941). Those ratings were combined into syndromes and then related to child behavior.

Despite that landmark work and other calls for observational approaches to avoid reliance on parents' self-reports (e.g., Merrill, 1946), parent observations did not become common until the 1960s (see the review by Lytton, 1971). Observational methodologies are increasingly being utilized, in part as the methodological issues and techniques are identified and discussed in the literature (e.g., Bakeman & Gottman, 1986; Cairns, 1979; Cousins & Power, 1986; Lamb, Suomi, & Stephenson, 1979).

Although some of the most influential observational studies have used observer ratings (e.g., Baumrind, 1971), the behavioral unit approach has been used far more often. This approach can be illustrated with Holden's (1983) observations of mothers and their 2-year-old children in the supermarket. This location was selected to observe naturally occurring parent-child interactions because of the challenging nature of the setting: mothers were there to shop, but also had to manage their children in the presence of all the tempting objects. As a result, it was expected that mothers would exhibit strategies for maintaining control of their children. Mothers used a variety of responses to child misbehavior, and conditional probability analyses of the sequential data helped to reveal that certain maternal "reactive control" techniques were more effective in achieving child compliance than others (e.g., diverting the child's attention was more effective than ignoring the child). However, the observations also revealed that mothers were using a second type of management behavior, which was labelled "proactive control" behavior. These intentional actions included initiating conversation with the child, giving the child food or objects, assigning the child a shopping task, or even avoiding certain aisles that contained tempting objects. A significant negative correlation was found between the rates of maternal initiating conversation and the rate of child misbehavior ($r[24] = -.58$, $p < .01$).

Besides the increase in naturalistic, home observations (e.g., Power, & Chapieski, 1986), an alternative trend of observational studies has been to bring parents into a laboratory in order to assess child rearing under more controlled conditions. Some laboratory observational studies have been designed to assess rates and types of parental behavior such as teaching, play, or controlling behaviors in relatively normal conditions (e.g., Brody, Pillegrini, & Sigel, 1986; Kuczynski, 1984), whereas in other studies, analog situations have been created in the laboratory. For example, Holden and West (1989) modeled the supermarket situation by bringing mothers and their young children to the laboratory where there were some tempting but "off-bound" objects as well as some mundane, non-tempting, objects that the children could play with. Mothers participated in three 8 min sessions: a control session and a "proactive" and a "reactive" session (the last two sessions were counter-balanced). Children engaged in more acceptable play and less off-bound play in the proactive session than in the reactive session. Results of that manipulation confirmed the causal nature of the correlation found in the supermarket observations: Mothers in the proactive control session had children who behaved better than when they were in the reactive control session. Such a demonstration required observational data and the ability to manipulate the setting afforded by a laboratory.

Combining Tools. Very few child-rearing instruments utilize both an observation and an interview. The best example of such an instrument is the Home Observation for the Measurement of the Environment

Inventory (HOME), developed by Bradley and Caldwell (1976) to measure the amount of stimulation the child is exposed to. The HOME consists of 45 items, about 2/3 of which rely on observations made by the experimenter (e.g., "Mother spontaneously vocalizes to child at least twice during visit"). The remaining items depend on the parent's verbal response to a question (e.g., "Mother reports that no more than one instance of physical punishment occurred during the past week"). Responses are coded as: Yes, No, or No information. The HOME takes about an hour to administer; it is indicative of the desire of many researchers for quick assessment tools that the format has recently been revised and reduced into a 30-item questionnaire that takes only 15 minutes for the parent to fill out (Frankenburg & Coons, 1986).

General evaluation of the tools. Some evaluative comments about the three types of methods for measuring child rearing are in order. A thorough evaluation would require a separate chapter; below, a brief discussion of advantages and disadvantages will serve to highlight some of the reasons why the measurement of child rearing is so difficult. Given specific instruments vary considerably within each type of method, it is somewhat harzardous to make such general comments—but only somewhat.

Parent questionnaires have two important attributes: speed of completion and privacy. No other approach can consistently boast of such quick access to data. One study has pertinent information (Holden & Edwards, 1989). Mothers were timed as they responded to a parent attitude survey of average length (51 items). On average, it took mothers 8 min to answer all the questions (range = 5-13 min). The investigator then was rewarded with four subscales.

The second key attribute of questionnaires is that they are typically filled out in privacy. This is particularly important when the questions are sensitive in nature, and thus, the parent may experience some evaluation apprehension concerning the experimenter's response. As Yarrow (1963) pointed out, parents are "extremely ego-involved reporters" (p. 217). By allowing the parent to fill-out the survey in private, the likelihood of this type of bias is reduced. The privacy attribute also allows the parent to fill out the survey in the privacy of their home and at their leisure. Given the hectic schedule that is a common byproduct of parenthood, this economy of time is clearly a major advantage of the method.

Despite the extensive role that parent questionnaires have played in

measuring child rearing, they have only rarely been subject to evaluation. However, there is plenty of fodder for criticism with such
instruments. Holden and Edwards (1989) have identified a number of
serious methodological and conceptual problems inherent in them.
Among the shortcomings: (a) decontextualized, global statements do
not map on to how parents think about their children; (b) vague and
ambiguous items are interpreted in different ways by different parents; (c) most questionnaires have limited or unknown psychometric
properties (i.e., reliability and validity); and (d) the static, unidirec-
tional model of parent-child interaction is inaccurate and does not
reflect current knowledge about parent-child relations.

The interview is a more complex method than a questionnaire
because data collection occurs in the context of a social interaction. As
such, there are advantages and disadvantages. In contrast to the
rigidity of a survey, the interview format usually allows for probes of
the parents' responses in a way that provides much more complete
and thorough information. The social situation inherent in the interview also enables the sensitive interviewer to recognize and correct
misunderstandings and persist in soliticiting answers to all the questions. However, the interview also requires face-to-face interactions
where the parents often feel (either justly or otherwise) that either they
or their children are being evaluated. The consequent evaluation
apprehension is liable to result in at least subtle biases in parental
reports. Hoffman (1957) pointed out that there are at least three
potential sources of error from interview data: forgetting, deliberate
withholding or falsifying information; and unconsciously motivated
omissions or distortions. These problems are not insurmountable
though, and he advised interviewers to direct questions to recently
occurring parental behavior, focus on details and specifics, and avoid
value judgements. Other limitations of the interview approach
include that it requires some skill on the part of the interviewer to
build rapport with a parent and it is more time consuming and
difficult to reduce into data than a questionnaire.

Observations represent a very different methodology because typically, someone other than the parent is doing the observing and
reporting. Thus, the data are behaviorally based and generally avoid
the possible contamination associated with parents' self reports. One
exception occurs when parents are trained to be the observers (e.g.,
Zahn-Waxler, Radke-Yarrow, & King, 1979). Through enlisting parents
as "research assistants", direct observations can be made when it
would not be otherwise possible due to the low rate of occurrence of

target behaviors or the effect of the observer on the parent's or child's behavior.

Although observation data generally avoids the self-report bias, such data can reflect *behavioral self-reports*. That is, when parents are aware that they are being observed, they may change their behavior toward a more socially accepted way. There is some data supporting this (e.g., Zegiob, Arnold, & Forehand, 1975). However, under certain circumstances, such as when a parent is over-loaded with tasks, such as shopping with a child, one can expect that the least of their worries is to try to impress the observer!

Problems also can occur in the reduction of observational data. As Ritter and Langlois (1988) have cleverly demonstrated, codings done at the molar but not molecular level are susceptible to bias. This is parallel to the warnings of distortion or potential sources of error in ratings of behavior in contrast to the use of behavioral units (Merrill, 1946). Ratings require a considerable amount of cognitive processing on the part of the observer, as Cairns and Green (1979) have pointed out, but may be more useful for describing the outcomes of development than systematic observations using behavioral units.

As these comments have highlighted, each method has advantages and disadvantages. To some extent, the methods used are dictated by the theoretical orientation, particular research questions, availability of instruments, and pragmatic considerations. It is unfortunate that one cannot purchase the one state-of-the-art tool to measure child rearing, but the phenomenon is too complex and multifaceted. Given there is no one correct approach, the burden is on the researcher to determine the optimal methods and measures for each particular study. We will now examine the match between research question and methods used by reviewing the literature on child rearing and prosocial development in children. To set the stage, we will summarize the proposed theoretical links between parental behavior and children's prosocial behavior.

Child rearing and children's prosocial behavior: Proposed links

There is wide accord among social development researchers that parents can influence the expression of prosocial behavior in their children through a variety of mechanisms. Based on recent reviews (e.g., Brody & Scaffer, 1982; Radke-Yarrow, Zahn-Waxler, & Chapman, 1983; Radke-Yarrow & Zahn-Waxler, 1986), four types of child-rearing mechanisms have been identified. These are: (a) the parent as model of prosocial behaviors; (b) parental control and teaching techniques; (c) affective relationships between parent and child; and (d) family structure and functioning.

The first child-rearing mechanism proposed to influence children's prosocial behavior is *modeling* the parent. Sigmund Freud, as is well known, believed that children acquired their conscience or superego through the identication with the same sex parent. Over the past 20 years, the concept of identification has given way to the more parsimonious explanation of modeling. Current social learning theorists would argue that if a child observes the parent to show empathy or be concerned about the welfare of others then the parent's child would be more likely to do so as well. The more competent, powerful, and warm the model is perceived by the child to be, the more likely the child is to model that parent's behavior (Moore & Eisenberg, 1984).

The second mechanism, that of *parental discipline and teaching*, received considerable attention in the 1950s and 1960s. The line of reasoning was that parental discipline appeared in early moral encounters where children, being egocentric, have to learn to consider the feelings and needs of others. It has long been thought that parental use of inductive reasoning contributes to children's prosocial behavior by prompting children to internalize the norm of considering others. On the other hand, authoritarian or power assertive disciplinary responses can undermine prosocial behavior (Moore & Eisenberg, 1984). As the child grows older, the parent may use more direct instruction, moral exhortations, and preaching. Discipline can be used to discourage behavior and thoughts that are morally unacceptable and instead, instill in children "a set of moral standards and values that provide the basis for self-controlled behavior" (Brody & Shaffer, 1982, p. 32). Positive reinforcement of a child's prosocial actions would fit in here. A further example of parental teaching lies in parental attributions. Parents' attributions about the source of their children's prosocial behavior is also thought to influence the children. If parents attribute prosocial actions to internal causes, children are more likely to be prosocial on subsequent opportunities as has been shown in the laboratory (e.g., Grusec & Redler, 1980).

The quality of the parent's *affective relationship* with the child is the third general mechanism considered to be an important contributor to prosocial behavior. As Hoffman (1979) has summarized, affection or nurturance is regarded as "important because it makes the child more receptive to discipline, more likely to emulate the parent, and emotionally secure enough to be open to the needs of others" (p. 958).

The last mechanism has been labelled *family structure and functioning*. It refers to less direct influences on prosocial development, such as family structure (e.g., number of children), communication, and relationships in the family. In particular, distribution of responsibilities (e.g., caregiving for a younger sibling or a pet) and the types of experiences the parent exposes the child to (e.g., attending church, visiting a sick friend in the hospital) are presumably relevant to prosocial development.

Child rearing and children's prosocial behavior: A methodological review

How adequately has the extant literature measured these four types of child-rearing mechanisms? To answer that question, we examined studies that have assessed child rearing and prosocial development. Studies were located by a computer search and from review articles on prosocial behavior (Brody & Shaffer, 1982; Feshbach, 1978; Hoffman, 1963; Moore & Eisenberg, 1984; Radke-Yarrow, et al., 1983; Radke-Yarrow & Zahn-Waxler, 1986). Through these sources, we assembled a set of 16 primary research reports where some assessment of child rearing was made. We assume the sample is representative of the literature.

The first question we examined was what are the methods used to measure child rearing? Three studies (Bryant & Crockenberg, 1980; LaVoie & Looft, 1973; Parikh, 1980) used two methods; the rest relied on only one. The most common method was the parent interview; nine or 56% of the studies included a maternal interview to quantify child rearing. Most of the interviews took the form of individual maternal interviews, but two included family discussions (LaVoie & Looft, 1973; Parikh, 1980). The use of parent questionnaires was the second most used approach, with six or 38% of the studies using some type of survey. Giving surveys to children to assess their perceptions of their parents' child rearing was the third most common approach, used in two of the 16 studies. Some type of observation was used in only two studies (Bryant & Crockenberg, 1980; Zahn-Waxler, et al., 1979). Table 1 lists the frequency with which each approach was used and the sample sizes and age of children used in the studies.

We next review the particular variables used to measure child rearing. The types of child-rearing variables assessed and the

Table 1   *Methods and some characteristics of studies relating child rearing and prosocial or moral development*

Methodology	Parent Sample	Ages of child
Parent Interview		
Burton, et al. (1961)	77 parents	4-year-olds
Grinder (1962)	140 mothers	5-6 through 11-12 year-olds
Hoffman (1963)	22 mothers	4-5 year-olds
LaVoie & Looft (1973)*	80 mother-father dyads	14-16 year-old boys
Hoffman (1975)	80 mother-father dyads	10-year-olds
Hoffman & Saltzstein (1967)	129 mothers, 75 fathers	12 year-olds
Mussen et al. (1970)	62 mothers	11 year-olds
Bryant & Crockenberg* (1980)	50 mothers	9-10 year-olds
Parikh (1980)*	40 mother-father dyads	13 & 15-year-olds
Parent Questionnaire		
LaVoie & Looft (1973)*	80 mother-father dyads	14-16 year-old boys
Gutkin (1975)	120 mothers	6, 8, & 11 year olds
Leahy (1981)	58 fathers, 70 mothers	15 year-olds
Olejnik & McKinney (1973)	78 mother-father dyads	4-year-olds
Parikh (1980)*	40 mother-father dyads	13 & 15-year-olds
Peterson, et al. (1984)	84 parents	3, 6, 12 year-olds
Child Questionnaire		
Eisenberg-Berg & Mussen (1978)	no parents (72 students)	14-17 year-olds
Rutherford & Mussen (1968)	no parents (63 boys)	4-year-old boys
Observations		
Bryant & Crockenberg* (1980)	50 mothers	9-10 year-olds
Zahn-Waxler, et al. (1979)	16 mothers	15 & 20 month-olds through 24-29 months

* – Used two methods to assess child rearing.

frequency across studies is listed in Table 2. The measures can be grouped into two categories: assessments of child-rearing behaviors in general, and assessments of parents' orientation to prosocial behavior, including their own and their children's.

Table 2   Number of studies that assessed particular child-rearing variables
related to prosocial and moral development

Variable	Number of studies
Child-Rearing Attitudes & Practices	
Disciplinary responses	10
Child-rearing practices (e.g., feeding, toilet training)	6
Nurturance, warmth, & affection	6
Degree of communication	1
Parental response to prosocial situations & issues	
Attitudes (re: cooperation, competitiveness, children's prosocial behavior)	4
Moral Reasoning & intentionality	3
Generosity and Altruism	2
Parents' empathy	1
Response to children when children are viewing persons in distress	1

As can be seen, parental discipline has been most commonly assessed.
In fact, in 10 out of the 16 studies, some type of assessment of parental
discipline was made. Parent attitudes toward or use of discipline has
been measured with each type of methodology. For example, in the
earliest study we identified that measured child rearing, Burton,
Maccoby, and Allinsmith (1961) interviewed mothers of 4-year-old
children to determine their disciplinary practices and level of warmth.
A few years later, Hoffman and Saltzstein (1967) interviewed fathers
as well as mothers. Their interview consisted of posing hypothetical
child-rearing situations to the parent. The use of a survey was
illustrated by Gutkin (1975) who instructed mothers to fill out a
questionnaire that contained stories of child misbehavior varying on
the dimensions of intentionality and amount of damage. The mothers
then indicated their likelihood to punish their children. Only one
study has used observational procedures to determine parental use of
discipline. Zahn-Waxler and her colleagues (1979) trained mothers to
observe and record both their own and their children's response to
incidences related to prosocial development.

The second most frequently assessed quality of parenting has been
non-disciplinary child-rearing practices. Six studies reported on child-
rearing behaviors such as socialization pressures (e.g., early weaning
and toilet training; Grinder, 1962) or parental supervision (e.g.,

encourages independence, offers protection; Leahy, 1981). Eisenberg-Berg and Mussen (1978) examined parental influence on empathy in adolescence by having 9, 11, and 12th grade students complete the 91-item Child Rearing Practices Report Q-Sort (Block, 1965) concerning their mothers' and their fathers' child-rearing attitudes and behavioral intentions.

Six studies have assessed a third quality of parenting: nurturance and warmth. These have been assessed with interview and survey measures. For example, Rutherford and Mussen (1968) used surveys to determine boys' perceptions of paternal warmth and nurturance. Hoffman (1975) took a different approach and measured parental affection by asking each parent to report retrospectively on how often he/she engaged in each of 16 behaviors (e.g., hugging, kissing) when the child was 5 or 6 years old.

Eleven of the studies, rather than looking at general qualities of child rearing, focused on parental responses or attitudes towards prosocial situations. Parental attitudes to their children's expression of prosocial behavior was measured in five studies. For example, Peterson, Reaven, and Homer (1984), examined parents' attitudes concerning their child's prosocial behavior. Various helping and sharing opportunities were presented on a questionnaire and parents were asked to make decisions about the situations in which they would want their children to behave prosocially. Other studies have measured prosocial behavior in the parents themselves, such as the parents' level of moral reasoning, empathy, or generosity.

Methodological issues

In reviewing this sample of studies designed in part, to assess how child rearing influences prosocial development, four types of methodological concerns can be raised. The first problem is one of omission. Of the four mechanisms which are thought to influence children's prosocial development, only one—that of parental disciplinary control—has been assessed frequently. And all but one of the assessments of discipline have relied on self-reported disciplinary behavior. Affective relationships have received attention in six studies, but again those are based on self-report measures. The mechanisms of modeling and family structuring have not received much attention. Thus, there has not been an adequate sampling of the parents' behaviors that might influence prosocial development. As Radke-

Yarrow, et al. (1983), point out, "Among the dimensions of rearing that are thoroughly missed in research are the content and nature of family discourse about human events and relationships" (p. 514).

A related point is the need to sample more than one quality of parental behavior. Though one parent may exhibit the "right" type of discipline, they have display the "wrong" type of warmth or fail to model prosocial behavior. Only by assessing multiple parental variables and, if necessary, controlling for variables, could that potential problem be addressed.

A second issue is inadequate attention directed toward the psychometric properties of the instruments used. None of the studies cite any validity data for their measures. Though such evidence is not needed for the two observational studies, some validation of instruments, particularly the questionnaires, is needed. Three studies use the Child Rearing Practices Report, an instrument whose psychometric properties have not been established adequately (Holden & Edwards, 1989). In contrast to the lack of validity data, all but five of the studies reported on some type of reliability: whether it be the coherence of subscales on questionnaires, or interrater codings of interview or observation data. In general, these assessments indicated acceptable levels of reliability, with only one exception (Grinder, 1962).

The third concern with these studies is in the sampling. Although most studies have good sample sizes (median = 78 parents), and have sampled parents' of children aged 15 months through 17 years (see Table 1), the parents have tended to have homogeneous characteristics. Of the ten studies that specify the race, seven use Caucasian parents. Of the 11 studies that specify socio-economic status, seven studies use parents from only the middle or upper-middle class, two studies contain lower-middle or working class parents, and two studies contain parents with a mixture of socio-economic backgrounds. Just one published study was conducted outside of America (Parikh, 1980). A more comprehensive sampling of parents from different backgrounds is needed to reveal more fully the range of parental behavior.

A fourth concern with these studies is the failure to examine explicitly the processes or mechanisms involved in relating childrearing behavior to prosocial development. The one exception is the study by Zahn-Waxler, et al. (1979), who examined the behavioral sequences that occurred follow incidents that could elicit prosocial behavior. Such process-oriented studies can help to reveal how one or more child-rearing variables influence behavior.

Common pitfalls in measuring child rearing

The above review prompts us to generate a list of common pitfalls or errors that occur in measurement of child rearing.

1. *Over-reliance on self-report data.* As reviewed above, the vast majority of instruments designed to assess parental behavior rely on self reports. The problem is not in self-reports, per se. It is in the incomplete knowledge we have about the quality of that data. If we were convinced of the accuracy of self-report data, such data would not be a methodological concern. Most efforts at measuring child rearing are guilty of this self-report problem; only 12% of the studies reviewed above utilized observational data.

2. *Inadequate attention to methodological issues.* This failure comes in various forms: the paucity of methodological critiques, the absence of studies comparing different methodologies, and inadequate attention to the psychometric properties of instruments in specific. For example, despite the widespread use of parental attitude questionnaires, the critique by Holden and Edwards (1989), is the first to appear, since the more limited critique of one attitude survey by Becker and Krug (1965). All too few methodological studies exist, such as comparisons between the quality of parental questionnaire, interview, and observational measures (e.g., Sears, 1965, Smith, 1958; Radke-Yarrow & Zahn-Waxler, 1979). Methodological work is not glamorous, but it is intrinsic to the study of child-rearing behavior.

3. *Over-emphasis on parental reactions, not actions.* When child rearing is studied, the attention is most often devoted to parental reactions to children at the expense of the study of nonreactive modes of influence (Radke-Yarrow & Zahn-Waxler, 1986). This problem has plagued much of the parent-child research literature, as is illustrated by the vast number of studies on parental disciplinary techniques. As Holden (1983) has shown, parental disciplinary responses are only part of child management. The rest of the story, and possibly the more important part, consists of anticipatory and other parental behaviors designed to preempt the need for discipline. In the case of prosocial development, most attention has been devoted to parental discipline with parental positive actions that could influence prosocial behavior, such as enrolling the child in a church school, rarely assessed. A recent study by Ladd and Golter (1988) showing how parents manage their preschooler's peer rela-

tions is exemplary of an effort to quantify how parental actions can influence children's social development.

4. *Static variables are used for a bidirectional, dynamic process.* Various social development researchers have advocated a focus on interactions and the use of interactive variables, rather than static type variables (e.g., Gewirtz, 1969; Sears, 1951). Instead, most investigators have relied on "one-sided", trait-like variables. Similarly, parents have been conceptualized as trait-like and unchanging; there is a need to study parents in more of a developmental way (Maccoby, 1984). When one recognizes that the parent-child dyad represents a complex relationship, and that there are many ways and levels by which that relationship can be described and studied (Hinde, 1976), then it is clear that current assessments of child rearing manage to describe only the "tip of the iceberg". Though it is easier to measure parents when they are conceived of as trait-like and unchanging, the accuracy of such a view must be questioned.

5. *Absence of replication studies.* In the area of parent-child relations, there are too few replication studies. For example, Baumrind's (1971) classic study of patterns of parental behavior has not been reproduced by other investigators, despite the prominence and importance of her findings. Though replication studies can be found in social development (e.g., Baldwin & Skinner, 1989), they are rare.

Directions for the measurement of child rearing

Despite the current problems in assessing child rearing, accurate and comprehensive assessments of child rearing can be collected. Toward that end, we provide three suggestions: one conceptual, one methodological, and one statistical.

The first requirement toward meeting the goal of improved assessment of child-rearing behavior involves sharpening our conceptions of parents and our measurement variables. Parental behavior is not trait-like and determined simply by global attitudes but is situationally sensitive and often characterized by considerable variability (e.g., Grusec & Kuczynski, 1980). Holden and Ritchie (1988) have suggested that parental social cognition is often characterized by conflicts and dilemmas about how they should behave, rather than a unitary attitude. Other researchers too have called for a more multi-dimensional view of parents (e.g., Radke-Yarrow, et al., 1983).

A clearer conceptualization of parents would also include a more comprehensive description of their relationships with their children. It would account for parental actions, as well as reactions, by revealing the role that parents play as "child-rearing executives". Parental activities such as organizing, structuring, administrating, anticipating, decision-making, and problem-solving need to be explicated. It would also include measurements of the different levels of analysis that characterize relationships. Hinde and Stevenson-Hinde (1986) identify eight dimensions of relationships or interactions, concerning: the content, the quality, the relative frequency and patterning, the reciprocal or complementary nature; the intimacy; the committment; the diversity; and interpersonal perception. Only some of these characteristics have been extensively studied in parent-child relations.

Our second suggestion focuses on methodology. Despite the fact that observations provide the cornerstone of a science (Hartup, 1978), researchers will always have to continue to rely on parental self-report data. Three reasons will suffice: much important behavior occurs when observers are unlikely to be present, to try to observe infrequently occurring behaviors would be prohibitively expensive, and interpersonal perception or social cognition can only be accessed by self reports. Therefore, the task is not to discard or abandon self-report data, the challenge is to understand it. This means to study what background variables or personality characteristics are associated with veridical reporting of behavior, identifying the conditions that are conducive to more accurate reports, under what conditions, and with what type of question or instrument is what needs to be studied.

In an effort to develop a new self-report device that is less susceptible to bias from being in an interview, but is more flexible and interactive than the reflective questionnaire methodology, Holden (1988) has been developing interactive software designed to probe parental social cognition and child-rearing self reports. The approach, labelled "computer-presented social situations", involves having parents individually respond to a coherent series of situations presented on a micro-computer. Among its advantages: it affords privacy and confidentiality; it is engaging to the participants; it allows for flexibility and branching; and it can simulate child-rearing situations and elicit more reflexive than reflective responses due to the interactive capabilities of computers.

One example of work currently underway utilizing this approach concerns assessing the accuracy of maternal self reports about their behavior. Using the techniques developed previously (Holden, 1983), mothers are being followed as they shop in the supermarket with their two-year-old children. About a week later they come to a psychology laboratory to operate a computer simulation of shoppping with their child. The simulation models the experience of shopping with a child, and eight different incidents of child misbehavior are presented. Mothers then select their most likely responses. The data analysis then involves examining the correspondence between mothers' observed behavior and their self-reported behavior. We expect that mothers will be accurate reporters for salient behavior—such as power assertive responses—but not accurate for other types of behaviors. We also expect that mothers who are more self-aware (as determined by a personality questionnaire), will have greater correspondence between the two sources of data than mothers who are less conscious of their behavior.

Our third suggestion for future work goes hand in hand with the first two suggestions. Given the multidimensional nature of parents and influences on children's development, more sophisticated statistical and conceptual approaches need to be developed and disseminated. Examples of these which will prove to be helpful in understanding child rearing include the social relations model (Kenny & La Voie, 1984), log-linear analyses (Bakeman & Gottman, 1986), and structural equation modeling and path analyses (e.g., Baldwin & Skinner, 1989; Belsky, Hertzog, & Rovine, 1986). Only through the use of more advanced multivariate statistical methods can we better tease apart and reveal the nature and consequences of parent-child relations.

Conclusion

We have argued that the degree of difficulty in studying child rearing has been underestimated. Unlike some other scientific enterprises where a sophisticated tool awaits the researcher, no one tool exists to provide a comprehensive assessment of child rearing. Rather, researchers must engage in complex calculations involving costs, benefits, and trade-offs in deciding on the method or methods to use. Considerations include such variables as the availability and quality of an instrument to assess child rearing, potential sources of bias, and the time requirements of the parent and researcher. As new conceptualizations of parents, knowledge of the qualities and characteristics of methods and instruments, and resources for measuring and analyzing child rearing are developed, researchers will gain greater freedom in the selection of methodologies. In turn, this will afford a greater understanding of how child-rearing practices affect development. One of the forefathers of the study of how children develop was the behaviorist John B. Watson. In 1928, he argued that the most difficult profession was child rearing. But Watson was wrong. The most difficult profession is measuring those who rear children.

References

Bakeman, R., & Gottman, J. M. (1986). *Observing interaction: An introduction to sequential analysis.* New York: Cambridge University.

Baldwin, A. L., Kalhoun, J., & Breese, F. H. (1945). Patterns of parent behavior. *Psychological Monographs, 58* (3).

Baldwin, D. V., & Skinner, M. L. (1989). Structural model for antisocial behavior: Generalization to single-mother families. *Developmental Psychology, 25,* 45-50.

Baumrind, D. (1971). Current patterns of parental authority. Developmental Psychology Monographs, 4 (1, Pt. 2).

Becker, W., & Krug (1965). The parent attitude research instrument—A research review. *Child Development, 36,* 329-365.

Belsky, J., Hertzog, C., & Rovine, M. (1986). Causal analyses of multiple determinants of parenting: Empirical and methodological advances. In M. E. Lamb, A. L. Brown, & B. Rogoff (Eds.), *Advances in developmental psychology, Vol. 4* (pp. 153-202). Hillsdale, NJ: Erlbaum.

Block, J. H. (1965). *The Child-Rearing Practices Report (CRPR): A set of Q items for the description of parental socialization attitudes and values.* Berkeley: University of California, Institute of Human Development.

Block, J. H., Block, J., & Morrison A. (1981). Parental agreement-disagreement on child-rearing orientations and gender related personality correlates in children. *Child Development, 57,* 712-721.

Bradley, R. H., & Caldwell, B. M. (1976). Early home environment and changes in mental test performance in children from 6 to 36 months. *Developmental Psychology, 12,* 93-97.

Brody, G. H., Pillegrini, A. D., & Sigel, I. E. (1986). Marital quality and mother-child and father-child interactions with school-aged children. *Developmental Psychology, 22,* 291-296.

Brody, G., & Shaffer, D. (1982). Contributions of parent and peers to children's moral socialization. *Developmental Review, 2,* 31-75.

Bryant, B., & Crockenberg, S. (1980). Correlates and dimensions of prosocial behavior: A study of female siblings with their mothers. *Child Development, 51,* 529-544.

Burton, R., Maccoby, E., & Allinsmith, W. (1961). Antecedents of resistance to temptation in four-year-old children. *Child Development, 32,* 689-710.

Cairns, R. B. (1979). *The analysis of social interactions: Methods, issues, and illustrations.* Hillsdale, NJ: Erlbaum.

Cairns, R. B., & Green, J. (1979). How to assess personality and social patterns: Obsevations or ratings? In R. B. Cairns (Ed.), *The analysis of social interactions: Methods, issues, and illustrations* (pp.209-226). Hillsdale, NJ: Erlbaum.

Champney, H. (1941). The measurement of parent behavior. *Child Development, 12,* 131-166.

Cousins, R. C., & Power, T. G. (1986). Quantifying family process: Issues in the analysis of interaction sequences. *Family Process, 25,* 89-105.

Crase, S. J., Clark, S. G., & Pease, D. (1979). *Iowa Parent Behavior Inventory manual.* Ames, IA: Iowa State University.

Eisenberg-Berg, N., & Mussen, P. (1978). Empathy and moral development in adolescence. *Developmental Psychology, 14* (2), 185-186.

Feshbach, N. (1978). Studies of empathetic behavior in children. *Progress in Experimental Personality Research, 8,* 1-47.

Frankenburg, W. K., & Coons, C. E. (1986). Home screening questionnaire: Its validity in assessing home environment. *Journal of Pediatrics, 108,* 624-626.

Gewirtz, J. L. (1969). Levels of conceptual analysis in environment-infant interaction research. *Merrill-Palmer Quarterly, 15,* 7-47.

Goldin, P. C. (1969). A review of children's reports of parent behaviors. *Psychological Bulletin, 71,* 222-236.

Grinder, R. (1962). Parental childrearing practices, conscience and resistance to temptation of sixth-grade children. *Child Development, 33,* 802-820.

Grusec, J., & Kucyznski, L. (1980). Direction of effect in socialization: A comparison of the parent vs. the child's behavior as determinants of disciplinary techniques. *Developmental Psychology, 6,* 1-9.

Grusec, J. E., & Redler, E. (1980). Attribution, reinforcement, and altruism. *Developmental Psychology, 16,* 525-534.

Gutkin, D. (1975). Maternal discipline and children's judgments of moral intentionality. *Journal of Genetic Psychology, 127,* 55-61.

Hartup, W. (1978). Levels of analysis in the study of social interaction: An historical perspective. In M. E. Lamb, S. J. Suomi, & G. R. Stephenson (Eds.), *Social interaction analysis: Methodological issues* (pp. 11-32). Madison, WI: University of Wisconsin.

Hinde, R. A. (1976). On describing relationships. *Journal of Child Psychology and Psychiatry, 17,* 1-19.

Hinde, R. A., & Stevenson-Hinde, J. (1986). Relating childhood relationships to individual characteristics. In W. W. Hartup & Z. Rubin (Eds.), *Relationships and development* (pp. 27-50). Hillsdale, NJ: Erlbaum.

Hoffman, M. (1957). An interview method for obtaining descriptions of parent-child interaction. *Merrill-Palmer Quarterly, 3,* 76-83.

Hoffman, M. (1963). Parent discipline and the child's consideration for others. *Child Development, 34,* 573-588.

Hoffman, M. (1975). Altruistic behavior and the parent-child relationship. *Journal of Personality and Social Psychology, 31,* 937-943.

Hoffman, M. (1979). Development of moral thought, feeling, and behavior. *American Psychologist, 34,* 958-966.

Hoffman, M., & Saltzstein, H. (1967). Parent discipline and the child's moral development. *Journal of Personality and Social Psychology, 5,* 45-57.

Holden, G. W. (1983). Avoiding conflict: Mothers as tacticians in the supermarket. *Child Development, 54,* 233-240.

Holden, G. W. (1988). Adults' thinking about a child-rearing problem: Effects of experience, parental status, and gender. *Child Development, 59,* 1623-1632.

Holden, G. W. (1990). Parenthood. In J. Touliatos, B. F. Perlmutter, & M. A. Straus (Eds.), *Handbook of family measurement techniques* (pp. 285-308). Beverly Hills: Sage.

Holden, G. W., & Edwards, L. (1989). Parent attitudes toward child rearing: Instruments, issues, and implications. *Psychological Bulletin, 106,* 29-58.

Holden, G. W., & Ritchie, K. (1988). Child rearing and the dialectics of parental intelligence. In J. Valsiner (Ed.), *Child development within culturally structured environments: Vol. 1, Parent cognition and adult-child interaction* (pp. 30-59). Norwood, NJ: Ablex.

Holden, G. W., & West, M. J. (1989). Proximate regulation by mothers: A demonstration of how differing parental styles affect young children's behavior. *Child Development, 60,* 64-69.

Kenny, D. A., & La Voie, L. (1984). The social relations model. In L. Berkowitz (Ed.), *Advances in experimental social psychology* (Vol. 18, pp. 141-182). New York: Academic.

Kucyznski, L. (1984). Socialization goals and mother-child interaction: Strategies for long-term and short-term compliance. *Developmental Psychology, 20,* 1061-1073.

Ladd, G. W., & Golter, B. S. (1988). Parents' management of preschooler's peer relations: Is it related to children's social competence? *Developmental Psychology, 24,* 109-117.

Lamb, M. E., Suomi, S. J., & Stephenson, G. R. (1979). *Social interaction analysis: Methological issues.* Madison: University of Wisconsin.

LaVoie, J., & Looft, W. (1973). Parental antecedents of resistance-to-temptation behavior in adolescent males. *Merrill-Palmer Quarterly, 19,* 107-116.

Leahy, R. (1981). Parental practices and the development of moral judgments and self-image disparity during adolescence. *Developmental Psychology, 17,* 580-594.

Lytton, H. (1971). Observation studies of parent-child interaction: A methodological review. *Child Development, 42,* 651-684.

Maccoby, E. (1984). Socialization and developmental change. *Child Development, 55,* 317-328.

Merrill, B. (1946). A measurement of mother-child interaction. *Journal of Abnormal and Social Psychology, 9,* 37-49.

Moore, B., & Eisenberg, N. (1984). The development of altruism. *Annals of Child Development, 1,* 107-174.

Mussen, P., Rutherford, E., Harris, S., & Keasey, C. (1970). Honesty and altruism among preadolescents. *Developmental Psychology, 3,* 169-194.

Olejnik, A., & McKenney, J. (1973). Parental value orientation and generosity in children. *Developmental Psychology, 8,* 311.

Parikh, B. (1980). Development of moral judgment and its relation to family environmental factors in Indian-American families. *Child Development, 51,* 1030-1039.

Peterson, R., Reaven, N., & Homer, L. (1984). Limitations imposed by parents on children's altruism. *Merrill-Palmer Quarterly, 30*(3), 269-286.

Power, T. G., & Chapieski, M L. (1986). Childrearing and impulse control in toddlers: A naturalistic investigation. *Developmental Psychology, 22,* 171-275.

Radke-Yarrow, M., & Zahn-Waxler, C. (1979). Observing interaction: A confrontation with methodology. In R. B. Cairns (Ed.), *The analysis of social interactions: Methods, issues, and illustrations* (pp. 37-66). Hillsdale, NJ: Erlbaum.

Radke-Yarrow, M., & Zahn-Waxler, C. (1986). The role of familial factors in the development of prosocial behavior: Research findings and questions. In D. Olweus, J. Block, & M. Radke-Yarrow (Eds.), *Development of antisocial and prosocial behavior* (pp. 207-233). New York: Academic.

Radke-Yarrow, M., Zahn-Waxler, C., & Chapman, M. (1983). Children's prosocial dispositions and behavior. In E. M. Hethington (Ed.), *Handbook of child psychology, Vol. 4,* 469-546.

Ritter, J. M., & Langlois, J. H. (1988). The role of physical attractiveness in the obsevation of parent-child interactions: Eye of the beholder or behavioral reality? *Developmental Psychology, 24,* 254-263.

Roehling, P. V., & Robin, A. L. (1986). Development and validitation of the Family Beliefs Inventory: A measure of unrealistic beliefs among parents and adolescents. *Journal of Consulting and Clinical Psychology, 54,* 693-697.

Rutherford, W. & Mussen, P. (1968). Generosity in nursery school boys. *Child Development, 39,* 755-765.

Schaefer, E. S., & Bell, R. Q. (1958). Development of a parental research instrument. *Child Development, 29,* 339-361.

Sears, C. (1899). Home and school punishments. *Pedagogic Seminary, 6,* 159-187.

Sears, R. R. (1951). A theoretical framework for personality and social behavior. *American Psychologist, 6,* 476-483.

Sears, R. (1965). Comparison of interviews with questionnaires for measuring mothers' attitudes toward sex and aggression. *Journal of Personality and Social Psychology, 2,* 37-44.

Sears, R., Maccoby, E., & Levin (1957). *Patterns of child rearing.* Evanston, IL: Harper & Row.

Smith, H. T. (1958). A comparison of interview and observation measures of mother behavior. *Journal of Abnormal and Social Psychology, 57,* 278-282.

Watson, J. B. (1928). *Psychological care of infant and child.* New York: Norton.

Yarrow, M. R. (1963). Problems of methods in parent-child research. *Child Development, 34,* 215-226.

Zahn-Waxler, C., Radke-Yarrow, M., & King, R. (1979). Child rearing and children's prosocial initiations toward victims of distress. *Child Development, 50,* 319-330.

Zegiob, L. E., Arnold, S., & Forehand, R. (1975). An examination of observer effects in parent-child interactions. *Child Development, 46,* 792-800.

CHAPTER 2

*N. Eisenberg & P. A. Miller**

The Development of Prosocial Moral Reasoning in Childhood and Mid-Adolescence

Until relatively recently, the study of moral development was primarily the study of anti-social or immoral behavior. Aggression, dishonesty, inability to resist temptation, and other undesirable behaviors were the topics of concern, whereas positive behaviors were relatively ignored. However, in the late 1960s and early 1970s, behavioral scientists started to turn their attention to the development of positive behaviors. This change in focus was undoubtedly related in part to a shift in the spirit of the times. The late 1960s was a time during which the general public became more concerned about long-standing injustices suffered by minorities and women, and American participation in an "unjust war" (the Vietnam War). These events lead to protests, liberalization of laws, and wider acceptance of humane values. It was in this atmosphere that behavioral scientists concentrated more of their efforts on trying to understand the development of humane behavior.

The emphasis on negative rather than positive moral behaviors was reflected in research on moral judgment as well as moral behavior. In specific, most of the research on moral reasoning until the mid 1970s was based on Kohlberg's (1969/1976) schema of moral reasoning and his interview materials. The central issues in the hypothetical dilem-

---

* Support for the preparation of this chapter was provided by grants from the National Science Foundation (BNS-8807784), the National Institute for Child Health and Development (K04 HD00717) and the National Institute of Mental Health (K02 MH000903) to the first author.

mas used in this research generally are justice and prohibition-related issues (i.e., laws, rules, punishments, disobeying an authority or his/her dictates, or living up to formal obligations) (Eisenberg-Berg, 1979). In none of Kohlberg's standard dilemmas is altruism the primary focus; altruistic behavior, if an option at all, is embedded in a context in which prosocial action constitutes a violation of a prohibition.

In this chapter, cross-sectional and longitudinal research concerning moral reasoning about prosocial issues are briefly reviewed. Our most recent data from a sample of adolescents in a longitudinal study will be emphasized. Then a preliminary model of prosocial moral reasoning is presented, along with empirical data that led to the construction of the model.

Prosocial Moral Reasoning: Age Trends

In our research on prosocial moral reasoning, we generally have used an interview technique similar to that of Kohlberg. The procedure in this research has involved presenting children or adolescents with several (usually four) prosocial dilemmas in an individual interview, and eliciting their reasoning regarding these dilemmas. Our dilemmas have differed from those of Kohlberg in that in each dilemma, the needs or wants of one individual are in direct conflict with those of another individual or group in a context in which the roles of prohibitions, punishments, authorities, and other formal criteria/obligations are irrelevant or minimized. An example of such a dilemma used with younger children (preschool and elementary-school aged) is as follows:

One day a girl (boy) named Mary (Eric) was going to a friend's birthday party. On her (his) way she (he) saw a girl (boy) who had fallen down and hurt her (his) leg. The girl asked Mary to go to her house and get her parents so the parents could come and take her to the doctor. But if Mary did run and get the child's parents, she would be late for the birthday party and miss the ice cream, cake, and all the games. What should Mary do? Why?

After each dilemma, children are asked what the story character should do and why. As for Kohlberg, our primary interest has been with the children's reasoning, not their choice of action.

Cross-Sectional Data

In several cross-sectional studies, the prosocial reasoning of American children aged 4 to 18 has been examined (e.g., Eisenberg & Shell, 1986; Eisenberg-Berg, 1979; Eisenberg-Berg & Neal, 1981). In these studies (as in others), children's interview responses were coded into a variety of categories, many of which resemble aspects of Kohlberg's stages (examples of most categories are in Table 1).

Table 1   Frequently Used Prosocial Moral Reasoning Categories[1]

1. *Obsessive and/or magical view of authority and/or punishment:* Avoidance of punishment and unquestioning deference to power are valued in their own right. The physical consequences of action determine its goodness regardless of human values and needs. Example: "If he didn't help, someone would find out and punish him."

2. *Hedonistic reasoning.*

   (a) *Pragmatic, hedonistic gain to the self:* Orientation to gain for oneself (besides gain resulting from direct reciprocity). Example: "She wouldn't help because she'd want to go to the party."

   (b) *Direct reciprocity:* Orientation to personal gain due to direct reciprocity (or lack of it) from the recipient of an act. Example: "She'd help because they'd give her food the next time she needed it."

   (c) *Affectional relationship:* Individuals' identifications with another, their liking for the other, and the other's relation to ones's own needs are important considerations in the individual's moral reasoning. Example: "She'd share because she'd probably have friends in the town."

3. *Nonhedonistic pragmatism:* Orientation to practical concerns that are not directly related to either selfish considerations or the other's need. Example: "I'd help because I'm strong."

4. *Concern for others' needs (needs-oriented reasoning).*

   (a) *Concern for others' physical and material needs:* Orientation to the physical and material needs of the other person. Examples: "He needs blood," or "She's hurt."

(b) *Concern for others' psychological needs:* Orientation to the psychological needs and affective states of the other person. Example: "They'd be happy if they had food."

5. *Reference to and concern with humaness:* Orientation to the fact that the other is human, living, a person. Example: 'He'd help because "they're human," or "they are people, too."'

6. *Stereotyped reasoning.*

   (a) *Stereotypes of a good or bad person:* Orientation to stereotyped images of a good or bad person. Example: 'A child would help because "it's nice."'

   (b) *Stereotyped images of majority behavior:* Orientation to "natural" behavior and what most people would do. Example: "It's only natural to help."

   (c) *Stereotyped images of others and their roles:* Orientation to stereotyped images of others and what others do. Example: "I'd help because farmers are nice people."

7. *Approval and interpersonal orientation:* Orientation to others' approval and acceptance in deciding what is the correct behavior. Example: "They'd like her if she helped."

8. *Overt empathic orientations.*

   (a) *Sympathetic orientation:* Expression of sympathetic concern and caring for others. Examples: "We would feel sorry for them," "She'd be concerned."

   (b) *Role-taking:* The individual takes the perspective of the other and explicitly uses this perspective in his or her reasoning. Examples: "I'my trying to put myself in his or her shoes," or "She'd know how it feels."

9. *Internalized affect.*

   (a) *Simple internalized positive affect and positive affect related to consequences:* The individual simply states that he or she would feel good as a result of a particular course of the consequences of his or her act for the other person. The affect must be used in a context that appears internalized. Example: "She'd help because seeing the villiagers fed would make her feel good."

(b) *Internalized positive affect from self-respect and living up to one's values:* Orientation to feeling good as the result of living up to internalized values. Example: "I'd feel good knowing that I had lived up to my principles."

(c) *Internalized negative affect over consequences of behavior:* Concern with feeling bad or guilty due to the consequences of an act. Example: "She would feel guilty because the girl was hurt."

(d) *Internalized negative affect due to loss of self-respect and/or not living up to one's values:* Orientation to feeling bad as the result of not living up to internalized values. Example: "He'd think badly of himself if he didn't do the right thing."

10. *Other abstract and/or internalized types of reasoning.*

(a) *Internalized law, norm, and value orientation:* Orientation to an internalized responsibility, duty, or need to uphold the laws and accepted norms or values. Examples: "She has a duty to help needy others," or "He'd feel he had a responsibility to assist because of his values."

(b) *Concern with the rights of others:* Orientation to protecting individual rights and preventing injustices that violate another's rights. Example: "I'd help because her right to walk down the street was being violated."

(c) *Generalized reciprocity:* Orientation to indirect reciprocity in a society (i.e., exchange that is not one-to-one but eventually benefits all). Example: "If everyone helps one another, we'd all be better off."

(d) *Concern with the condition of society:* Orientation to improving the society or community as a whole. Example: "If everyone helps, society would be a lot better."

---

1 *Less frequently used categories such as those related to equality of individuals and social contract are omitted. See Eisenberg (1977) and Eisenberg-Berg, 1979. Adapted from Eisenberg-Berg, 1979.*

To briefly summarize our findings, in the cross-sectional research we have found that older preschoolers and young elementary-school children use little authority and punishment-oriented reasoning to justify moral decisions; rather, they verbalize much hedonistic reasoning and needs-oriented reasoning (primitive empathic reasoning in which they merely orient to or label the other's need). In elementary school, children's judgments begin to reflect approval-oriented considerations, and the desire to behave in stereotypically "good" ways. In contrast, high school students sometimes make judgments reflecting abstract principles, internalized affective reactions (e.g., guilt or positive affect) related to living up to one's principles, and/or self-reflective empathic modes of reasoning reasoning (e.g., sympathetic, role taking, positive affect/consequences, negative affect/consequences reasoning). These more advanced modes of reasoning are used in addition to other less advanced modes (such as hedonistic, needs-oriented, stereotypic, and approval-oriented reasoning), with developmentally less mature, self-oriented modes of reasoning such as hedonism being used especially to justify decisions not to assist (see Eisenberg, 1982, 1986, for reviews).

Only one of our cross-sectional studies has involved elementary-school *and* high school students. In this particular study, students in grades 2, 4, 6, 9, 11, and 12 were interviewed using our prosocial moral dilemmas. Multivariate linear trend analyses were used to examine age trends across the entire group in the types of reasoning used to justify prosocial decisions. Categories of reasoning that increased with age included reference to and concern with humanness, role taking, positive affect/consequences, positive affect/self-respect and living up to one's own values, negative affect/consequences, internalized law, norm, and value orientation, concern with rights of others, generalized reciprocity, and concern with the condition of society. Stereotypic reasoning related to good/bad people or behavior and approval/interpersonally-oriented reasoning decreased in use with age. In addition, when considering reasoning both for and against assisting, a primary focus on self-related hedonistic reasoning decreased with age. Finally, although needs-oriented reasoning was used by students of all ages, only younger students used primarily this mode of reasoning (Eisenberg, 1977; Eisenberg-Berg, 1979).

Longitudinal Data: Trends from Preschool to the End of Elementary School
In several longitudinal followups of the preschool children in one of our early studies, we have further delineated developmental changes

in children's prosocial moral judgment (Eisenberg, Lennon, & Roth, 1983; Eisenberg, Miller, Shell, McNalley, & Shea, 1991; Eisenberg, Pasternack, & Lennon, 1984; Eisenberg, Shell, Pasternack, Lennon, Beller, & Mathy, 1987; Eisenberg-Berg & Roth, 1980). Children who initially were aged approximately 4-5 have been reinterviewed 1 1/2, 3, 5, 7, 9, and 11 years later. Moreover, a second small cohort of 4-5 year-olds who were started a year after the primary cohort also has been reinterviewed repeatedly (Eisenberg et al., 1987). At all follow-ups, groups of children who had not been previously tested have been interviewed to assess the effects of repeated testing on moral reasoning.

There are a few interesting patterns of findings for moral reasoning during the preschool and elementary school years that are not evident when trend analyses include data for adolescents as well as elementary school children. Thus, I first briefly discuss the findings for the analyses up until sixth grade (published in Eisenberg et al., 1987), and then present data from two more recent followups during the adolescent years (Eisenberg et al., 1991).

The results of the longitudinal followups generally have been consistent with the cross sectional work. Across the preschool and elementary school years, hedonistic reasoning dropped in frequency of use from age 4-5 until mid-elementary school age, at which time it leveled off in use. Simultaneously, there was significant increase in needs-oriented reasoning, which leveled off by age 9-10 years. The use of a number of other categories of reasoning increased during the elementary school years: pragmatic reasoning, approval/interpersonal reasoning, stereotypes of good and bad persons, and direct reciprocity reasoning. Moreover, three relatively sophisticated categories of reasoning (role taking, sympathy, and positive affect related to consequences of one's behavior for others) were used significantly more at age 11-12 than at younger ages, although the linear increases in sympathetic and role taking reasoning held only for girls. Girls also used significantly more role taking reasoning than boys. Thus, in the late elementary school years, other-oriented types of prosocial reasoning seemed to be emerging more rapidly for girls than for boys (Eisenberg et al., 1987).

The results for the younger, smaller cohort have been very similar to those for the primary cohort. Moreover, children interviewed for the first time at the various followups have not differed much in reasoning from the primary cohort; thus, there has been little evidence of an effect from repeated testing.

Longitudinal Data: Trends from Preschool Age Through Mid-Adolescence
In the last two longitudinal followups, the children in the primary
cohort were 13-14 and 15-16 years of age. No children in this cohort
have been lost from the study from age 11-12 to age 15-16. Of the 37
original subjects, 32 were interviewed at age 15-16.

To examine the recent data, multivariate and univariate analyses of
variance were computed with one with-subjects factor (time) and one
between subjects factor (sex). Based on these analyses, we found that
hedonistic reasoning decreased dramatically in the early elementary
school years, leveled out in usage until age 13-14, and then increased
slightly in use at age 15-16. Although the sex X quadratic trend was
not significant, it is interesting to note that the increase in hedonistic
reasoning in mid-adolescence was only for boys.

An inverse pattern was found for needs-oriented reasoning. It
increased dramatically in use in the early school years, leveled off in
use, and then decreased somewhat in adolescence.

Direct reciprocity reasoning increased in use until age 11-12, and
then decreased in mid-adolescence. Similar patterns were also
obtained for stereotypic and approval-oriented reasoning; they
increased in frequency until age 13-14 and then declined in use.

Affectional relationship reasoning was verbalized less than the
other modes of reasoning, and its pattern of change was less clear. Use
of affectional relationship reasoning increased and decreased somewhat until mid-adolescence, at which time it increased considerably.
Pragmatic reasoning, which seemed to reflect in part students' consideration of aspects of the concrete situation, increased in frequency
with age.

Some modes of reasoning did not emerge until at least 9 to 10 years
of age (role taking, sympathetic, positive affect about the consequences of one's behavior). Both role taking and positive affect/
consequences reasoning were used more frequently with age. In
addition, girls used somewhat more role-taking reasoning ($p < .07$)
than did boys.

Several other categories of reasoning were used with any real
frequency only in adolescence. For example, categories of reasoning
that seemed to emerge around age 13 to 14 were positive affect/self-
esteem, negative affect/consequences, internalized norm and law, and
equality of individuals reasoning. Both internalized norm and positive affect/self-esteem reasoning were used increasingly with age
from early to mid-adolescence. Similarly, reasoning about generalized
reciprocity—the notion that helping others increases the likelihood

that other will assist yet other people and that everyone benefits—which was virtually never verbalized until age 15-16, increased in use with age in early to mid-adolesence.

In summary, the results of our recent analyses of the longitudinal data are fairly consistent with the cross-sectional data. Hedonistic reasoning generally decreased in use with age, although it increased somewhat in use for 15-16 year old boys. Needs-oriented reasoning increased in early childhood, leveled off in use, and then decreased in use with age. Direct reciprocity reasoning, approval-oriented reasoning, and stereotypic reasoning all increased with age in the elementary school years and then started to decrease with age. The more mature modes of reasoning that were used with any frequency—role taking, positive affect/consequences, positive affect/self-esteem, internalized norm, and generalized reciprocity—emerged in late elementary school or thereafter, and their use increased with age into adolescence.

Levels of Prosocial Moral Reasoning
Based on both the cross-sectional and the earlier phases of the longitudinal research described above, we delineated an age-related sequence of development of prosocial moral judgment. These levels are presented in Table 2. The lowest level (reflecting hedonistic, self-oriented reasoning) has been found to be dominant in the reasoning of only preschool and elementary school children; Levels 4b and 5 (internalized values and related affect) predominate in the reasoning of only a minority of high school students. However, individuals do not reason exclusively at one level, or even at a given level and the adjacent levels. As was mentioned previously, adolescents occasionally verbalize Level 1 reasoning when justifying the decision not to assist (Eisenberg-Berg, 1979), although most reason primarily at levels 2, 3, or 4.

Our recent longitudinal data primarily raise some questions about our levels of prosocial moral reasoning. For example, direct reciprocity reasoning, which is in our lowest level, increases significantly with age in elementary school and then is used somewhat less frequently by adolescents. In a study with German and American children, an increase in direct reciprocity reasoning in the elementary school years also was observed (Eisenberg, Boehnke, Schuhler, & Silbereisen, 1985). This type of reasoning clearly involves cognitive concepts of exchange and relationships between people, and is more sophisticated cognitively than merely a focus on what the self desires (e.g., hedonistic reasoning). However, although this type of reasoning increases with

Table 2   Levels of Prosocial Reasoning *

Level 1. Hedonistic, self-focused orientation: The individual is concerned with self-oriented consequences rather than moral considerations. Reasons for assisting or not assisting another include consideration of direct gain to the self, future reciprocity, and concern for others because one needs and/or likes the other (due to affectional tie.) (Predominant mode primarily for preschoolers and younger elementary-school children).

Level 2. Needs-oriented orientation: The individual expresses concern for the physical, material, and psychological needs of others even though the other's needs conflict with one's own needs. This concern is expressed in the simplest terms, without clear evidence of self-reflective role taking, verbal expressions of sympathy, or reference to internalized affect such as guilt. (Predominate mode for many preschoolers and many elementary-school children).

Level 3. Approval and interpersonal orientation and/or stereotyped orientation: Stereotyped images of good and bad persons and behaviors and/or considerations of other's approval and acceptance are used in justifying prosocial or nonhelping behaviors. (Predominant mode for some elementary and high-school students.)

Level 4a. Self-reflective empathic orientation: The individual's judgements include evidence of self-reflective sympathetic responding or role taking, concern with the other's humannedd, and/or guilt or positive affect related to the consequences of one's actions (predominant mode for a few older elementary-school children and many high-school students).

Level 4b. Transitional level: The individual's justifications for helping or not helping involve internalized values, norms, duties, or responsibilities, concern for the condition of the larger society, or refer to the necessity of protecting the right and dignity of other persons; these ideas, however, are not clearly and strongly stated. (Predominant mode for a minority of people high-school age or older.)

Level 5. Strongly internalized stage: Justifications for helping or not helping are based on internalized values, norms, or responsibilities, the desire to maintain individual and societal contractual obligations or improve the condition of society, the belief in the dignity, rights, and equality of all individuals. Positive or negative affect related to the maintenance of self-respect for living up to one's own values and accepted norms also characterizes this stage. (Predominant mode for only a small minority of high school students and no elementary-school children.)

* Reprinted from Eisenberg, 1986

age, it clearly reflects concern with one's own outcomes. Thus, it has been left in the lowest level of reasoning, although it now clear that these levels reflect conceptions regarding morality, and not just empirical, age-related changes in reasoning.

Another example of a finding that is difficult to explain is the increase in the low level affectional relationship reasoning in adolescence. However, a number of the adolescents who were coded as using this type of reasoning were merely inquiring whether the needy other was a friend or relative, and this type of reasoning may have been relatively insignificant in their final reasoning. In addition, this mode of reasoning was used rather infrequently overall, in part because our dilemmas explicitly involve the helping of people who are not likely to be friends or relatives. If we were to examine reasoning about helping known others, the pattern for affectional relationship reasoning might look very different.

The trends for approval/interpersonal-oriented reasoning and sterotypic good/bad reasoning help to explain a prior contradiction in the empirical literature. Eisenberg-Berg (1979), in a previously cited cross sectional study, found decreases in these types of reasoning over the elementary and high school years. In contrast, in our longitudinal data for elementary children, we had found that these types of reasoning were used increasingly with age. The data from the latest longitudinal followups clarify these inconsistencies; the aforementioned modes of reasoning appear to increase in frequency in the elementary school years and then are used less in mid-adolescence.

Gender Differences in Prosocial Moral Reasoning
In the analysis of the longitudinal data from preschool to grade 6, we had found that there were some gender differences in the use of other-oriented, self-reflective modes of reasoning (Eisenberg et al., 1987). Girls used more role-taking reasoning, and the use of sympathetic and role-taking reasoning seemed to emerge in late elementary school for girls but not boys. This pattern of findings seemed consistent with our earlier finding of gender differences favoring females in certain higher level, often empathic, modes of reasoning, including reference and concern with humanness and sympathetic orientation (Eisenberg, 1977). The earlier data also were consistent with Gilligan's (1982) assertion that females are more care-oriented than males in their moral orientations. However, according to the results of the adolescent followups, males and females differed relatively little in their moral reasoning (although females still were somewhat more likely to

use more role taking reasoning overall), and males appeared to catch up in regard to the emergence of sympathetic and role-taking reasoning. It will be interesting to see whether males and females differ in the use of higher level, self-reflective modes of reasoning as these modes of reasoning become more frequently used in later adolescence.

Socialization of Prosocial Moral Reasoning

Socialization experiences seem to play a role in the development of prosocial behavior (Eisenberg & Mussen, 1989; Radke-Yarrow, Zahn-Waxler, & Chapman, 1983); thus, it is reasonable to expect socialization to affect the development of prosocial moral reasoning. However, research concerning the socialization of prosocial moral reasoning is scarce. Nonetheless, it is possible to draw some tentative conclusions about socialization correlates from the existing literature.

At the age of 5 to 6 years, children's level of prosocial moral reasoning has been associated with supportive (but not especially affectionate), nonpunitive, nonauthoritarian child-rearing practices, combined with concern for the child's safety but not overrestriction of autonomous functioning. At age 7 to 8, children's level of moral reasoning has been correlated with maternal reports of nonrestrictive, nonpunitive child-rearing practices; however, this pattern of associations was relatively weak (Eisenberg et al., 1983). The relation between maternal report of child-rearing attitudes and practices appears to be even weaker at age 9-10 years. In one study in which the associations between children's moral reasoning and maternal warmth/conflict, overprotection, nonrestrictiveness with regard to emotional expression and auttonomy were examined, the only finding was a positive relation between maternal emphasis on autonomy and boys' level of prosocial moral reasoning (Eisenberg, Pasternack, & Lennon, 1984).

Despite the fact that the association between children's prosocial moral reasoning and maternal practices and attitudes seems to decline with age in the elementary school years, other data suggest that socialization variables are associated with adolescents' prosocial moral reasoning. High school females' reports of maternal emphasis on autonomy, achievement, and competition rather than overprotection have been positively related to higher level prosocial moral judgment, as have paternal coldness and father-daughter conflict. For males, there may be a modest relation between level of prosocial moral reasoning and maternal supportiveness and emphasis on the importance of autonomy and responsibility (Eisenberg, 1977). The latter results for males are consistent with the other data indicating that sociocognitive functioning in adolescence is enhanced by parental acknowledgment of the child as a separate person and parents' openness to the child's point of view (Grotevant & Cooper, 1986). An extra push toward individuation may be necessary for the female adolescent to develop her own perspective and reasoning (Grotevant & Cooper, 1986); maternal emphasis on competition and conflict between daughter and father may provide that push.

Based on the limited available data, it is difficult to draw any firm conclusions regarding changes with age in the pattern of relation between parental practices and children's prosocial moral reasoning. In the studies of younger children (Eisenberg et al., 1983, 1984), information regarding maternal practices was obtained from mothers. In the research involving adolescents (Eisenberg, 1977), data pertaining to parental practices were obtained from the students, not the parents. Thus, the fact that children's moral reasoning seemed to be more highly related to parental practices in adolescence than in mid-childhood might be due the fact that children's reports of parental practices were used in the study of adolescence. Consistent with this idea, Janssens, Gerris, and Janssen (1989) found that nine- to twelve-year-olds' reports of parental practices, but not parental reports of their own practices, were correlated with the children's prosocial moral reasoning.

The structure of the institutions to which the individual is exposed also appears to influence adolescents' level of prosocial moral judgment. For example, Higgins et al. (1984) found that students who attended a democratic high school with an emphasis on community used more and higher level social responsibility reasoning, and were more likely to report that they would make and act on prosocial decisions, than were students from regular schools. Apparently, the moral atmosphere of the school affected students' moral reasoning about prosocial moral issues.

In summary, based on the limited research, it appears to socialization experiences influence children's prosocial moral reasoning, although this influence may be limited in scope, especially at some ages. We will return to the issue of the role of socialization in prosocial moral reasoning later in this chapter.

Summary

In summary, our cross-sectional and longitudinal research with American children has lead us to identify fairly consistent patterns of development for prosocial moral reasoning. However, we are not claiming that our levels of reasoning are invariant in sequence or universal across cultures. Moreover, although our levels of moral reasoning do, to some degree, reflect age trends, philosophical conceptions regarding morality are also reflected in the levels, and socialization experiences appear to be associated with children's level of prosocial moral reasoning. We now deal with issues of this sort more extensively in the context of discussing a preliminary model of prosocial moral reasoning.

The Model

Our preliminary model of prosocial moral reasoning is illustrated in Figure 1. Briefly, in this model an individual's level of moral reasoning is viewed as reflecting his or her moral values, as well as other values, needs, and preferences. Moreover, moral reasoning is seen as limited by level of socio-cognitive development, and as influenced by situational and personality factors.

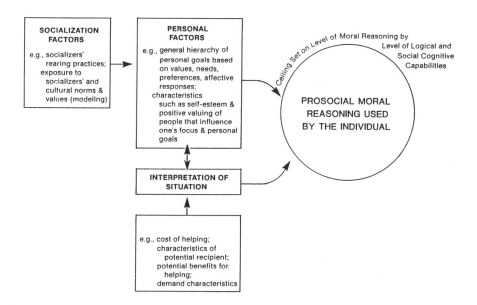

Figure 1 Factors affecting prosocial moral reasoning

More specifically, the individual's moral reasoning in a given context is viewed as an outcome of characteristics of the situation—the situation as interpreted by the individual. The individual's choice of reasoning also is influenced by his or her values and goals, which are, in turn, partly a function of socialization experiences and cultural factors. However, these goals and values, and the motivation to act in accordance with one's goals and values, are differentially activated in different contexts. Finally, sociocognitive factors play a role; level of abstract thinking, perspective taking, and related sociocognitive skills set a ceiling on the individual's prosocial moral reasoning.

The Role of Cognitive and Sociocognitive Capabilities

Several assumptions are inherent in this model. Some of these assumptions are similar to those of Kohlberg; some are not. According to Kohlberg and his colleagues (Colby, Kohlberg, & Kauffman, 1987), Kohlberg's stages of moral reasoning meet the criteria for "hard" structural stage models. In other words, each of his stages is viewed as being qualitatively different in structure from all other stages; the sequence of stages is invariant and universal; each stage is a "structured whole" (i.e., does not represent a specific response determined by knowledge and familiarity with that task or similar tasks but an underlying thought-organization); and each stage displaces or integrates the structures found at lower levels (i.e., stages are hierarchical integrations).

Based on his notion of "hard", qualitatively different stages, Kohlberg has asserted that development is limited, in part, by the individual's level of socio-cognitive development, that is, the complexity of the individual's cognition with regard to social phenomena. In Kohlberg's view, individuals who are at a low or moderate level with regard to logical and socio-cognitive functioning—often due to their young age and corresponding incomplete development—cannot be expected to understand or use higher level modes of moral judgment (Colby et al., 1987).

The assumption that there is a ceiling set on the individual's level of moral reasoning due to his/her level of logical and/or socio-cognitive development seems applicable to the domain of prosocial moral judgment. Young children clearly are incapable of expressing higher level modes of reasoning; level 4 or 5 reasoning—reasoning reflecting self-reflective role taking or empathy and internalized values or value-based emotional reactions—is relatively rare even among children in elementary school (e.g., Eisenberg-Berg, 1979; Eisenberg et al., 1983, 1987; Munekata & Ninomiya, 1985).

The Role of Social Factors

An assumption in our model that is somewhat at odds with Kohlberg's model is that socialization, including at the cultural level, has an important effect on individuals' moral reasoning. It does so not only by influencing opportunities for sociocognitive perspective-taking (the primary process mediating the effect of socialization on moral judgment in Kohlberg's model), but also by affecting the development and prioritizing of various goals, values, and needs. For example, other-oriented values and the importance of competition and achievement undoubtedly vary across cultures and subcultures. As is discussed soon, the relative importance of such goals and values often may be relevant to the individual's moral reasoning in a given context.

There are data consistent with our view that social factors influence moral reasoning—data from both studies of the relation of socialization practices to moral judgment and cross-cultural studies. As was discussed previously, parental emphasis on autonomous decision-making appears to affect level of moral judgment (Leahy, 1981; Eisenberg, 1977; Parikh, 1980), as does the degree to which an institutional setting (such as a school) encouraages participation in decision making (Higgins, Kohlberg, & Powers, 1984).

More impressive, however, are the cross-cultural and sub-cultural differences that are found in prosocial moral reasoning. Although there are few differences in the reasoning of children from American and German urban areas (Eisenberg, Boehnke, Schuhler, & Silbereisen, 1985) and the reasoning of Japenese students changes in ways similar to that of American students (Munekata & Ninomiya, 1985; Ninomiya, 1987), Fuchs, Eisenberg, Hertz-Lazarowitz, and Sharabany (1986) noted moderate differences in the moral reasoning of American city children, Israeli city children, and Israeli kibbutz children. In this study involving 55 American, 29 kibbutz, and 36 Israeli city children, two sets of analyses were computed: one in which the American data and those of the combined Israeli sample were compared, and one in which all three groups of third graders (American, Israeli city, and Israeli kibbutz) were compared.

According to the results, American children used much more physical needs-oriented reasoning (a relatively early emeraging, simple mode of other-oriented reasoning). In contrast, Israeli children verbalized more hedonistic, direct reciprocity, affectional relationship, humanness, role-taking, and internalized law/norm orientation reasoning. When the reasoning of the children from all three groups was compared, American children scored significantly higher on physical needs-oriented reasoning than did either kibbutz or Israeli city children. In contrast, kibbutz children used more concern with humanness and internalized law/norm orientation reasoning than did either American or Israeli city children, and Israeli city children verbalized more role taking reasoning than did either of the other two groups.

To summarize, the American children were especially likely to base their decisions on the relatively immature type of reasoning in which individuals simply orient to others' needs. In contrast, kibbutz children were more likely than other children to justify decisions with an appeal to the notion that the needy other was a "person" (with the implication, direct or implied, that people are special) or by referring to internalized norms, rules, or values. Both of these types of reasoning preferred by the kibbutz children are relatively mature developmentally and seem to reflect the ideological emphasis of the kibbutz.

Moreover, two of the self-oriented (i.e., hedonistic) types of reasoning that were used frequently by the Israeli children (direct reciprocity, affectional relationship) were used considerably (although not significantly) more by kibbutz children and are consistent with the emphasis on relationships and exchange among group members that is characteristic of a communal society. Finally, the fact that Israeli city children expressed somewhat more hedonistic reasoning (the difference between Israelis' and Americans' use of this category was primarily due to the high rate of hedonistic reasoning among Israeli city children) may be due to the emphasis on consumerism in Israeli cities, combined with the fact that many commodities are scarce or expensive.

Recently we conducted a three-year followup of the kibbutz and city Israeli children (Eisenberg, Hertz-Lazarowitz, Fuchs, & Sharabany, 1990). They were administered several moral dilemmas that were either identical or similar in theme to those administered when the children were in third grade. In response to these dilemmas, children verbalized more direct reciprocity and concern with humanness reasoning whereas the city children used more hedonistic and pragmatic reasoning. According to univariate analyses for these same categories of reasoning, use of direct reciprocity reasoning increased with age for both groups, but much more so for the Israeli kibbutz children. Pragmatic (nonmoral) reasoning increased in use for only the city children. As in the original study, it appeared that the differences in the kibbutz and city children's reasoning were consistent with their social environments. Consistent with the kibbutz ideology and communal life style, the types of reasoning expressed by the kibbutz children reflected concern with exchange with others in the group and with the importance of other human beings, whereas the types of reasoning used more by the city children were self-oriented or merely practical (not concerned with moral issues). Moreover, these findings are consistent with recent work in which kibbutz children's moral reasoning on Kohlberg's dilemmas was examined (Snarey, Reimer, & Kohlberg, 1985) and with other work in which researchers have found that kibbutz children display higher levels of prosocial behavior than do city Israeli children (see Fuchs et al., 1986, for a review).

Even more relevant are the data collected by Anne Tietjen (1986) from people in two isolated Maisin coastal villages, Uiaku and Ganjiga, Papua New Guinea. In these Maisin villages, the traditional social organization is strong; the people are tightly bound by kinship obligations. Moreover, the Maisin are collectivistic rather than individualistic in orientation.

Tietjen interviewed individuals using a slightly modified version of Eisenberg's stories. Sixty-nine children were interviewed in 1982; 34 of these children were reinterviewed in 1983. Eight adolescents and 24 parents also responded to stories.

According to the data, Maisin children as well as adolescents and adults used more physical needs-oriented reasoning than any other type of reasoning. Hedonistic reasoning was next most frequently used. The younger Maisin children's reasoning was similar to that of American children of comparable age in that physical needs-oriented and hedonistic reasoning were the most common modes of judgment, with the former being more prevalent than the latter. However, unlike for Americans, the reasoning of the older Maisin children and adults differed relatively little from that of the children. The most salient developmental changes were significant, modest increases in affectional relationship, sympathetic and psychological needs-oriented reasoning (especially the latter) with age. Hedonistic reasoning peaked in third grade (perhaps because of the initial effects of exposure to Western values) and dropped off somewhat thereafter. Authority and punishment reasoning was low at all ages, as was the use of higher level reasoning categories. In brief, although the moral judgment of the Maisin clearly fit the coding scheme of Eisenberg (there were no "new" types of reasoning noted by the coders), there are both similarities and clear differences between the reasoning of the Maisin and that of Americans in other research.

The fact that the Maisin adolescents and adults exhibited very little high level reasoning is consistent with the results of cross-cultural research concerning Kohlbergian moral judgment. Researchers (e.g., Nisan & Kohlberg, 1982; Turiel, Edwards, & Kohlberg, 1978; White, Bushnell, & Regemer, 1978; see Snarey, 1985) have found that people from non-Western, rural and nonindustrial societies exhibit relatively little higher level reasoning. However, in a small, face-to-face, traditional society such as that of the Maisin, it is reasonable that the types of reasoning used by the people reflect attention to others' needs (physical needs-oriented, psychological needs-oriented, and sympathetic reasoning), as well as concern with that which is possible for them to give to others (hedonistic and perhaps pragmatic concerns). A cooperative, other-oriented approach on the dyadic level is both necessary for the survival of such groups and highly valued.

In brief, we are arguing that the moral judgments of children reflect, to some degree, the values and concerns of the culture. Once children are capable of understanding a certain type of reasoning, differential use of that reasoning seems to be linked to the importance of the concerns embedded in the reasoning for persons in the society. Thus, cultural factors seem to affect choice of reasoning within that sphere of moral reasoning accessible to the individual.

Variation in Intraindividual Use of Prosocial Moral Judgment
Another assumption of our model is that within the range of prosocial moral reasoning accessible to a given individual, a variety of levels may be verbalized. Indeed, we frequently find that individuals' prosocial moral reasoning plummets when they decide against the prosocial action alternative. Our findings differ from those of Kohlberg; for him, the criterion of "structured wholeness" implied that much of an individual's moral reasoning is at a single level and that people do not use and/or have access to reasoning stages much below or above their dominant stage.

In part, differences in our data and those of Kohlberg regarding intraindividual variability seem to be due to differences in coding schemes. To some degree, Kohlberg and his colleagues have examined competence, not performance, in the domain of moral reasoning. Indeed, their coding system is designed to measure the most advanced or highest level reasoning that an individual uses with any consistency, not the entire range of reasoning verbalized by individuals in their moral reasoning. Indeed, Kohlberg's coding system includes several techniques that systematically exclude, to some degree, reasoning that varies greatly from that of the individual's dominant stage, especially lower level reasoning. For example, stages of reasoning that comprise less than 10% of the individual's reasoning are discarded when computing the person's composite score (Colby, Kohlberg, Gibbs, & Lieberman, 1983). In addition, if a lower level idea is expressed in a manner that is not viewed as being prescriptive (i.e., is not used as a moral justification), it is not coded. Finally, reasoning at lower levels is eliminated if the same basic idea or concern is also expressed in a more mature fashion. The rationale for this scoring rule is that the lower level reason is viewed as being conceptually consistent with the higher level reasoning, only expressed incompletely or inadequately (Colby, 1984).

The scoring system that has been used to code prosocial moral judgment differs in a variety of ways from that of Kohlberg. One important difference is that with the prosocial scoring system, *all* of the individual's reasoning is scored regardless of frequency of use and regardless of whether higher level reasoning concerning the same general idea is used (unless the reasoning is too incomplete to score). This is one reason why we do not find that stages are "structured wholes." As was noted previously, we, like Rest (1979), have found that individuals who are capable of higher level reasoning still may express much lower level reasoning. Thus, Kohlberg's criterion of hierarchical integration does not seem to apply to prosocial moral judgment, at least as we assess it.

As was noted previously, a basic assumption of my model is that the individual's choice of moral reasoning is influenced by his or her values and goals, including cultural and subcultural values and goals, as well as more individual preferences and values. For example, individuals who are concerned about social appearances and others' approval would be expected to use relatively high levels of approval/ interpersonally oriented reasoning whereas empathic persons with other-oriented value systems should tend to use whichever mode of empathic, other-oriented moral reasoning is appropriate for their age (e.g., needs-oriented reasoning for younger children; sympathetic or role-taking reasoning for older children). In contrast, those concerned with material gain should tend to use hedonistic reasoning, whereas the desire to behave in a manner condoned by society would be expected to be associated with stereotypic reasoning. In other words, the type of reasoning preferred by a given individual is expected to be a function of aspects of the person frequently labeled as components of "personality." These include the individual's value orientation and other characteristics such as degree of positive valuing of people, level of self-esteem, and degree of self-concern, all of which color the individual's needs, goals, and values. Put differently, although the individual's level of competence with regard to moral reasoning is limited by developmental factors, performance within one's sphere of competence is believed to be a function, in part, of individual differences on a variety of personal variables.

Although limited, there is some empirical support for this view. Among fourth and sixth graders, we have found that individuals concerned with presenting a socially desirable image tended to use relatively high levels of approval-oriented reasoning (Eisenberg et al., 1987). Similarly, American children who scored high on Bryant's (1982) empathy scale were found to use relatively high amounts of age-appropriate empathic modes of reasoning (needs-oriented reasoning for 2nd graders; sympathetic reasoning for 4th graders; see Eisenberg, 1986; Eisenberg et al, 1987). A similar relation between needs-oriented reasoning (psychological needs) and empathy scores has been noted among the Maisin in New Guinea (Tietjen, 1984).

Each person has a number of personal goals based upon personal values, needs and preferences (see Staub, 1978, 1984). As was noted by Staub (1978), in a given situation, several of these personal factors may be relevant to moral decision making. Moreover, various personal goals activated in a given context may conflict with one another. For example, in a situation in which a person could publically assist another at a cost to the self, the desire for social approval and/or empathically-based concerns may conflict with the desire to preserve one's own resources. In such a circumstance, the relative importance of the various relevant goals in the individual's hierarchy of personal goals should be reflected in his or her choice of moral justifications, as well as in the relative importance of various modes of reasoning (when more than one mode is used).

The role of the situation or context generally has been deemphasized in work on moral judgment, but the context surely affects which personal needs, values, and goals are likely to be salient when considering a specific moral dilemma. For example, children (Eisenberg-Berg, 1979) and adults (Sobesky, 1983) tend to use more lower level reasoning (e.g., hedonistic rather than needs-oriented) as the perceived cost of assisting another increases. In one study, children used more hedonistic reasoning and less other-oriented reasoning when they merely reasoned from their own perspective rather than that of a third person other (Eisenberg-Berg & Neal, 1981). This pattern of findings likely occurred because self-related goals and needs were more salient when reasoning from the first person perspective. Moreover, there is undoubtedly an interaction between situational and personal factors; which personal goals are salient in a specific situation for a given person will be a function, in part, of the configuration and specific content of the individual's values, needs, and goals. For example, the goal of obtaining others' approval will be elicited by somewhat different cues (e.g., by different degrees of public visability or the presence of different observers) for different persons. In addition, the individual's interpretation of a situation, including which aspects of the situation are apprehended, perceived as salient, and/or are distorted, is undoubtedly a function, in part, of personal characteristics. Indeed, it is unlikely that context alone is ever the sole influence on choice of moral reasoning within the individual's sphere of competence; even in extreme situations in which contextual influences are overwhelming (e.g., if the cost of behaving in a manner consistent with higher level reasoning were death), there would probably still be individual differences in the level of moral judgment expressed (e.g., consider Socrates' behavior and reasoning prior to his death).

Summary

To summarize, in this preliminary model of prosocial moral reasoning, socialization history and current situational factors have a marked influence on individuals' moral reasoning. Moreover, personality characteristics are much more salient in our model than in Kohlberg's. Finally, we want to specifically acknowledge that this is only a working model. It is not assumed that the factors that influence level of moral reasoning are limited to those in our model. Nonetheless, it is our view that the model is a useful heuristic when considering the variables that contribute to the individual's level of prosocial moral reasoning concerning moral conflicts in specific contexts.

References

Bryant, B. (1982). An index of empathy for children and adolescents. *Child Development, 53,* 413-425.

Colby, A. (1984). Personal communication.

Colby, A., Kohlberg, L., Gibbs, J., & Lieberman, M. (1983). A longitudinal study of moral judgment. *Monographs of the Society for Research in Child Development, 48* (Serial No. 200), 1-124.

Colby, A., Kohlberg, L., & Kauffman, K. (1987). Theoretical introduction to the measurement of moral judgment. In A. Colby L. Kohlberg (Eds.), *The measurement of moral judgment* (Vol. 1; pp. 1-75). New York: Cambridge Press.

Eisenberg, N. (1977). The development of prosocial moral judgment and its correlates (Doctoral dissertation, University of California, Berkeley, 1976). *Dissertation Abstracts International, 37,* 4753B. (University Microfilms No. 77-444, 184).

Eisenberg, N. (1982). The development of reasoning regarding prosocial behavior. In N. Eisenberg (Ed.), *The development of prosocial behavior.* New York: Academic Press.

Eisenberg, N. (1986). *Altruistic emotion, cognition and behavior.* Hillsdale, NJ: Erlbaum and Associates.

Eisenberg, N., Boehnke, K., Schuhler, P., & Silbereisen, R. K. (1985). The development of prosocial behavior and cognitions in German children. *Journal of Cross-Cultural Psychology, 6,* 69-82.

Eisenberg, N., Hertz-Lazarowitz, R., Fuchs, I., & Sharabanny, R. (1990). Prosocial reasoning in Israeli kibbutz and city children: A longitudinal study. *Merrill-Palmer Quarterly, 36,* 273-285.

Eisenberg, N., Lennon, R., & Roth, K. (1983). Prosocial development: A longitudinal study. *Developmental Psychology, 19,* 846-855.

Eisenberg, N., Miller, P.A., Shell, R., McNally, S., & Shea, C. (1991). Prosocial development in adolescence: A longitudinal study. *Developmental Psychology, 27,* 849-857.

Eisenberg, N., & Mussen, P. (1989). *The roots of prosocial behavior in children.* Cambridge, England: Cambridge University Press.

Eisenberg, N., Pasternack, J. F., & Lennon, R. (1984, March). *Prosocial development in middle childhood.* Paper presented at the biennial meeting of the Southwestern Society for Research in Human Development, Denver.

Eisenberg, N., & Shell, R. (1986). Prosocial moral judgment and behavior in children: The mediating role of cost. *Personality and Social Psychological Bulletin, 12,* 426-433.

Eisenberg, N., Shell, R., Pasternack, J., Lennon, R., Beller, R., & Mathy, R. M. (1987). Prosocial development in middle childhood: A longitudinal study. *Developmental Psychology, 23,* 712-718.

Eisenberg-Berg, N. (1979). Development of children's prosocial moral judgment. *Developmental Psychology, 15,* 128-137.

Eisenberg-Berg, N., & Neal, C. (1981). The effects of person of the protagonist and costs of helping on children's moral judgement. *Personality and Social Psychology Bulletin, 7*, 17-23.

Eisenberg-Berg, N., & Roth, K. (1980). The development of children's prosocial moral judgment: A longitudinal follow-up. *Developmental Psychology, 16*, 375-376.

Fuchs, I., Eisenberg, N., Hertz-Lazarowitz, R., & Sharabany, R. (1986). Kibbutz, Israeli city, and American children's moral reasoning about prosocial moral conflicts. *Merrill Palmer Quarterly, 32*, 37-50.

Gilligan, C. (1982). *In a different voice: Psychological theory and women' development.* Cambridge, MA: Harvard University Press.

Grotevant, H. D., & Cooper, C. R. (1986). Individuation in family relationships. *Human Development, 29*, 82-100.

Janssens, J. M. A. M., Gerris, J. R. M., & Janssen, A. W. H. (1989, April). *Childrearing, empathy and prosocial development.* Paper presented at the biennial meeting of the Society for Research in Child Development, Kansas City, MO.

Kohlberg, L. (1969). Stage and sequence: The cognitive-developmental approach to socialization. In D. A. Goslin (Ed.), *Handbook of socialization theory and research* (pp. 325-480). New York: Rand McNally.

Kohlberg, L. (1976). Moral stage and moralization: The cognitive- developmental approach. In T. Lickona (Ed.), *Moral development and behavior: Theory, research, and social issues* (pp. 84-107). New York: Holt, Rinehart, and Winston.

Leahy, R. (1981). Parental practices and the development of moral judgment and self-disparity during adolescence. *Developmental Psychology, 17*, 380-394.

Munekata, H., & Ninomiya, D. (1985). The development of prosocial moral judgments. *Japanese Journal of Educational Psychology, 33*, 157-164.

Ninomiya, K. (1987, July). Prosocial moral judgments in Japanese adolescents. Paper presented at the 9th biennial meetings of the International Society for the Study of Behavioral Development, Tokyo.

Nisan, M., & Kohlberg, L. (1982). Universality and variation in moral judgment: A longitudinal and cross-sectional study in Turkey *Child Development, 53*, 865-876.

Parikh, B. (1980). Development of moral judgment and its relation to family environment factors in Indian and American families. *Child Development, 51*, 1030-1039.

Radke-Yarrow, M., Zahn-Waxler, C., & Chapman, M. (1983). Prosocial dispositions and behavior. In P. Mussen (Ed.), *Manual of child psychology.* Vol. 4. *Socialization, personality, and social development* (E. M. Hetherington, Ed.) (pp. 469-545). New York: John Wiley & Sons.

Rest, J. R. (1979). *Development in judgment moral issues.* Minneapolis: University of Minnesota Press.

Snarey, J. R. (1985). Cross-cultural university of socio-moral development: A critical review of Kohlbergian review. *Psychological Bulletin, 97,* 202-232.

Snarey, J. R., Reimer, J., & Kohlberg, L. (1985). Development of social-moral reasoning among kibbutz adolescents: A longitudinal cross-cultural study. *Developmental Psychology, 21,* 3-17.

Sobesky, W. E. (1983). The effects of situational factors on moral judgments. *Child Development, 54,* 575-584.

Staub, E. (1978). *Positive social behavior and morality: Social and personal influences* (Vol. I). New York: Academic Press.

Staub, E. (1984). Steps toward a comprehensive theory of moral conduct: Goal orientation, social behavior, kindness and cruelty. In J. Gerwirtz & W. Kurtines (Eds.), *Morality, moral development, and moral behavior: Basic issues in theory and research* (pp. 241-260). New York: John Wiley & Sons.

Tietjen, A. (1984). Personal communication.

Tietjen, A. (1986). Prosocial reasoning among children and adults in a Papua New Guinea society. *Developmental Psychology, 22,* 861-868.

Turiel, E., Edwards, C. P., & Kohlberg, L. (1978). Moral development in Turkish children, adolescents, and young adults. *Journal of Cross- Cultural Psychology, 9,* 75-85.

White, C. B., Bushnell, N., & Regnemer, J. L. (1978). Moral development in Bohemian school children: A 3-year examination of Kohlberg's stages of moral development. *Developmental Psychology, 14,* 58-65.

J.M.A.M. Janssens & J.R.M. Gerris

Child Rearing, Empathy and Prosocial Development

During the past three decades Hoffman (1963, 1970, 1975, 1976, 1982) reported about children's prosocial development and about the way their parents can promote this development. One concern regarding prosocial development is the definition of prosocial behavior or altruism. Prosocial behavior or altruism means action on behalf of someone else that involves a net cost to the actor. Types of altruism or prosocial behavior are sharing, comforting or helping another in distress, and making a donation to someone in need. According to Eisenberg and Miller (1987), it is necessary to differentiate between altruism and prosocial behavior. Prosocial behavior is behavior that results in benefits for another, but the motive is unspecified. Altruism is voluntary behavior intended to benefit another, which is not performed with the expectation of receiving external rewards. In this study we focused on prosocial behavior.

Another aspect of prosocial development—also in this study—concerns prosocial moral reasoning, that is, reasoning about conflicts in which the individual must choose between satisfying his or her own wants or needs and those of others in context in which laws, punishments, authorities, formal obligations, and other external criteria are irrelevant or deemphasized (Eisenberg-Berg, 1979). Prosocial reasoning and prosocial behavior are probably related to each other, because this type of moral conflict elicits reasoning about actions that potentially benefit another at a cost to the self (Eisenberg-Berg & Hand, 1979).

The contribution of the parent to the child's prosocial development has not been a primary focus of interest in research on prosocial development (Hoffman, 1975). In this study we analyzed three child-rearing practices that can promote the child's prosocial development: child discipline, parental support, and demandingness. Hoffman (1963, 1970, 1975, 1982) emphasized the importance of parental discipline, i.e. parental behavior with the intent of directing the behavior of the child in a manner desirable to the parents. Hoffman (1970) and Rollins and Thomas (1979) distinguished three types of discipline; coercion or power assertion, induction, and love withdrawal. Coercion or power assertion is "behavior of the parent in a contest of wills, which results in considerable external pressure on the child to behave according to the parent's desires" (Rollins & Thomas, 1979, p. 321). For example, the parent punishes physically or deprivates the child from objects or privileges. Induction is behavior "with the intent of obtaining voluntary compliance to parental desires by avoiding a direct conflict of wills with the child" (Rollins & Thomas, 1979, p. 322). The parent gives explanations or reasons for desired behavior or points out the consequences of the behavior for the child or for others. Love withdrawal is parental behavior "indicating disapproval of the child's behavior" (Rollins & Thomas, 1979, p. 322). The parent ignores or isolates the child or he/she gives explicit indications of rejection or disappointment.

One major finding of Hoffman's research was that induction was positively and that power assertion was negatively related to prosocial development, whereas no relationship was found between love witdrawal and prosocial development. According to Hoffman (1970), the positive influence of induction was mediated by the child's empathy. Empathy is an affective state that stems from the apprehension of another's emotional state. According to Hoffman and Saltzstein (1967), induction motivates the child to pay attention to the victim's harm and/or distress. The realization that the child himself or herself is the cause of that harm or distress evokes an empathic response in the child. The child empathizes with the victim and is motivated to repair the harm or to relieve the distress. Induction may help the child to become aware of the victim's feelings, and thus help guide the child's future actions in an altruistic direction. Power assertion and love withdrawal on the other hand evoke anger or fear. As a result, the child does not focus on the victim's harm or distress, but on the negative consequences the transgression has for himself or herself (punishment or love withdrawal). Power assertion and love withdrawal promote an egoistic rather than a prosocial attitude.

Although Hoffman's explanation seems plausible, Radke-Yarrow, Zahn-Waxler, and Chapman (1983) concluded in their review that positive, negative and no associations have been found between power-assertive techniques and prosocial behavior. The same holds for relations between induction and prosocial development. A possible explanation for these contradicting results is that the consequences of power assertion or induction depend on the use of these techniques as part of a total pattern of parental characteristics and techniques. "If power assertion is linked negatively with children's prosocial behaviors, it is likely to be associated at the same time with negative attitudes on the part of the parent and, most likely, with punitive assertion... In the context of a positive and responsive parent power assertion may relate quite differently to prosocial behavior by children. The influence of induction on prosocial behavior is similarly modified by rearing context, particularly affective contextual factors" (Radke-Yarrow et al., 1983, p. 509-510). Staub (1979) also argued that patterns of parental practices rather than specific practices are important predictors for child development.

In these child-rearing patterns a supportive relation between parent and child seems to be important. Rollins and Thomas (1979) and Hoffman (1975) have emphasized the positive influence of parental support on the child's prosocial development. Rollins and Thomas defined support as "behavior manifest by a parent toward a child that makes the child feel comfortable in the presence of the parent and confirms in the child's mind that he is basically accepted and approved as a person by the parent" (Rollins & Thomas, 1979, p. 320). According to Hoffman (1963), support does not frustrate the child with unfulfilled needs that blinds the child to other's needs. Support would make the child feel secure and would minimize self-concern; it is not necessary to worry about his or her own needs and the child has the opportunity to consider the needs of others. Radke-Yarrow et al. (1983) pointed to a possible mediating function of empathy between parental support and prosocial development. In their view, support leaves room to consider the other's feelings and to empathize with others. However, Radke-Yarrow et al. (1983) concluded in their review that in some studies relations have been found between affection or warmth or nurturance and prosocial development, whereas in other studies no relations have been found. But in all these studies "nurturance has been dealt with as the parents' generally accepting and supportive behavior" (Radke-Yarrow et al., 1983, p. 505). According to Radke-Yarrow et al. (1983), it is possible to look more analytically into the child's experience for circumstances in which parental nurturance is especially critical. One such class of experiences may consist of situations in which the child is distressed. In these situations support means responsiveness; the parent is sensitive to the child's needs and feelings and reacts directly and adequately. The importance of parental responsive support was also emphasized by Staub (1979). When parents react responsively, the child feels that he/she controls the environment and that he/she can trust that environment. According to Staub (1979), these feelings of control and trust can focus the child on the needs of others.

Moreover, in this context we may consider it as critical that the child perceives the parental support as responsive (Staub, 1979). When the child perceives parental behavior as responsive, parental support promotes feelings of trust and control, and as a consequence, the child's focus on others' needs may be positively affected. In Hoffman's research (1970) many of the significant relations between child rearing and the child's prosocial and moral behavior pertained rather to the child's perception of child-rearing practices than to the parental practices as reported by the parents.

In later publications, Hoffman (1976, 1982) emphasized not only the importance of parental induction and support, but also the influence of parental behavior in which the parent makes an appeal to the child's responsibility. Other authors (Maccoby & Martin, 1983; Baumrind, 1971) called this parental behavior Demandingness. When parents are demanding, they make an appeal to responsibility, to mature behavior, to independence, or to the child's problem solving ability. Although in the last years the concept Demandingness is emphasized, one can find hardly any research about relations between demandingness and prosocial development. Maccoby and Martin (1983) reported only studies in which the influence of demandingness was studied in relation to responsiveness. They refered only to a study of Yarrow, Waxler, and Scott (1971). These authors found an interaction between nurturance and demandingness in the acquisition of prosocial behavior. Furthermore, it was concluded in Maccoby and Martin's review that parents who are demanding and responsive have children who are are more competent, more independent and more socially responsible. Eisenberg, Lennon, and Roth (1983) concluded that for children in elementary school encouragement of autonomy seems to be important for prosocial behavior and Staub (1979) concluded from Baumrind's studies that both encouragement of responsibility and independence are important for altruism.

From the review of Maccoby and Martin (1983), it is clear that it is difficult to draw conclusions about effects of demandingness without considering parental responsiveness. In some studies (Coopersmith, 1967) it was found that demandingness was related to parental support and control. Parents who set high standards for their children's competence and obedience and consistently enforce these standards tend to favor inductive over coercive methods and foster a democratic style of family decisions (Maccoby & Martin, 1983).

What can we conclude about relations between child rearing and prosocial development from the above mentioned studies? First, it seems important to study parental behavior as perceived by the child. Second, we have to consider all aspects of child rearing simultaneously when we study relations between child rearing and prosocial development. This procedure seems necessary when support, discipline and demandingness are interrelated. Following this line of reasoning, our first aim in this study was to analyze relations between these child-rearing concepts. Our second aim was to analyze relations between these concepts and prosocial development. Third, we investigated whether empathy is an intervening variable between child rearing and prosocial development.

There is evidence for an association between empathy and prosocial development on the one hand and between child rearing and empathy on the other. We already mentioned the mediating link of empathy between support and prosocial behavior. Support leaves room to consider the feelings of others and to empathize with them. Moreover, child-rearing practices in which the child is invited to or confronted with the distress of others (induction) and exhortations or demands for mature behavior (demandingness) can be considered as empathy provoking behaviors. According to Hoffman and Saltzstein (1967), induction motivates children to focus their attention on the harm done to others as the salient aspect of their transgressions, and thus to help integrate their capacity for empathy with the knowledge of the human consequences of their own behavior. Possibly the same may hold true for the influence of demandingness. When parents demand that their child has to consider the needs of others or when they teach the child that he/she is responsible to help another in need, they might promote their child's empathic capacities.

 When empathy is a mediating link between child rearing and prosocial development, relations must exist not only between child rearing and empathy, but also between empathy and prosocial development. Eisenberg and Miller (1987) found low to moderate positive relations between empathy and prosocial development, depending on the method used to assess empathy. Apparently, a positive relationship can be expected particularly when a self-report questionnaire is used. Such a self-report measure may be considered as an index for a person's dispositional empathy. In our study we used Bryant's empathy scale (Bryant, 1982).

Eisenberg and Miller mentioned several reasons for the moderate relations between empathy and prosocial development. One reason is that in most studies only one measure was used for prosocial development. In our studies we used several measures. First, we measured the child's prosocial moral reasoning. Second, we asked the teachers and classmates about the children's prosocial behavior. We not only related these measures to empathy and child rearing, but also we analyzed the relations between these measures.

 In summary, we tested the following model (Figure 1). In testing this model we also analyzed whether empathy was an intervening variable between child rearing and prosocial development or just an other dependent variable like prosocial development (Figure 2).

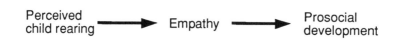

Figure 1 Prosocial development explained from child rearing with empathy as mediating variable

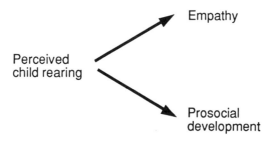

Figure 2 Prosocial development and empathy explained from child rearing

Method

Subjects
Data were obtained from 120 Dutch families; both parents and one child of each family participated. The sample consisted of 61 boys and 59 girls. The children's age was between 9;5 and 12;11. From the families 28% belonged to lower class, 50% to middle and 22% to upper class.

Instruments
Empathy. Empathy was assessed with Bryant's empathy scale (Bryant, 1982). This scale consisted of 22 items (nine-point scale). (e.g. "Sometimes I cry when I watch TV"). Scores varied between 22 and 198. The more a child reacted empathically, the higher the score. The reliability (Cronbach's alpha) in our reseach was .69.

Prosocial moral reasoning. Prosocial moral reasoning was assessed with four Eisenberg stories (the flood, swimming story, robbery story and the hospital) (Eisenberg-Berg, 1979). Each of these stories contained a conflict between the actor's own wants, needs, and desires and those of a needy other. The child was asked what he should do and why. The answers were audiotaped and transcribed verbatim. For each story we coded (inter rater reliability = .81):
a. whether the child used hedonistic reasoning when deciding to help or not to help others;
b. whether the child used need-oriented reasoning;
c. whether the child had an emphatic orientation or showed internalized affects.
Few children had an empathic orientation or showed an internalized affect. Therefore we decided to compute only one score for each child, the number of stories in which the child refered to the needs of others, to an empathic orientation or to internalized affect without any use of hedonistic reasoning. Scores varied between zero and four. The higher the score, the more the child tended to satisfy others' needs rather than his or her needs.

Prosocial behavior. To assess *prosocial behavior* we used three measures. First, we asked the teachers of the children to fill in Weir and Duveen's Prosocial Behaviour Questionnaire (Weir & Duveen, 1981). This questionnaire consisted of 20 items (six-points). Each item refered to the child's prosocial behavior in the classroom (e.g. "helps other children when are feeling sick"). Scores varied between 20 and 120. The higher the score, the more prosocial the child was in the classroom according to the teacher. The reliability of this scale (alpha) was .90. Second, we asked classmates to mention three children in their class whom they liked most, and three who helped most. For each child numbers of nominations by classmates as being most liked and as most helping were computed. These numbers were divided by the total number of children in the class, because the number of children in each class was different. The higher the score, the more the child was seen as prosocial by classmates.

Child rearing. To assess child rearing we interviewed the children. They were asked to imagine eight concrete situations in which a child transgressed a norm or rule and we asked them what their parents would do or say when they transgressed as the child in the story. An example is:

You play with wooden blocks together with a friend and you need some of the blocks your friend has. Your friend does not need these blocks, but he refuses to give them to you. You become angry and strike your friend. He starts to cry.

All answers were audiotaped and transcribed. To compute scores for support, discipline, and demandingness, we analyzed each answer and decided whether the parent was supportive, power assertive, inductive and/or demanding in a situation according to the child (inter rater reliability = .83). We coded an answer or a part of an answer as *supportive* when the parent would comfort the child or would show understanding for the child's transgression because it was elicited by another child. An answer or part of it was coded as *power assertive* when a parent would punish the child (physically or not) or would threaten with punishment. Behavior was coded as *inductive* when the parent would point at the consequences of child's transgression, or would ask the child to imagine how he/she would feel when he/she was the victim or when the parent would explain the situation or would give reasons not to transgress in the future. Finally, behavior was coded as *demanding* when the parent would point at the child's responsibility or would say which mature behavior he or she expected in such a situation. For each parent we computed four scores:

1. number of situations in which the child perceived behavior coded as supportive;
2. number of situations in which the child perceived behavior coded as power assertive;
3. number of situations in which the child perceived behavior coded as inductive;

4. number of situations in which the child perceived behavior coded as demanding.

According to their children parents rarely used love withdrawal. Therefore, we did not compute a score for this type of discipline.

Results

The first question of our research concerned the interrelations between child-rearing practices as perceived by the child. Relations between the four measures of perceived child rearing are presented in Table1 (mothers) and Table 2 (fathers). It appeared that maternal support, discipline, and demandingness were related to each other. Maternal support was positively related to induction, to demandingness and negatively to maternal power assertion. Demandingness was positively associated with induction and negatively with power assertion. Also induction and power assertion were negatively related to each other. Mothers who were supportive to their child were also more demanding, more inductive, and less power assertive.

Table 1   *Relations Between Measures of Perceived Mother's Child rearing*

	Support	Induction	Power assertion
Induction	.24*		
Power assertion	−.19*	−.53*	
Demandingness	.16*	.42*	−.50*

*$p < 0.05$

Table 2   *Relations Between Measures of Perceived Father's Child rearing*

	Support	Induction	Power assertion
Induction	.11		
Power assertion	−.27*	−.54*	
Demandingness	.08	.25*	−.57*

*$p < 0.05$

For fathers, we found a similar pattern of correlations (Table 2). Support, induction and demandingness were positively related to each other; however, only the correlation between induction and demandingness was statistically significant. Correlations between power assertion on the one hand and induction and demandingness on the other were significantly negative.

From Table 1 and Table 2 the conclusion may be drawn that for both parents demandingness and induction were positively related and that these two child-rearing practices were negatively related to power assertion. Maternal support was moderate positively associated with induction and demandingness and negatively with power assertion. Father's support, however was only negatively related to power assertion.

Our second question concerned relations between measures of prosocial development and empathy. These relations are presented in Table 3. It appeared that empathy was moderately, but significantly related to prosocial reasoning and being most liked by classmates. However, correlations between empathy and measures of prosocial behavior in the classroom (measured by teachers and classmates) were not significant. The school-related measures of prosocial development were related to each other. Children who were seen as prosocial by their teacher, were often most liked by their classmates and were seen as most helping by their classmates. Children who helped classmates were also more liked. A third finding from Table 3 concerned the positive relation between prosocial behavior and

Table 3   Relations Between Measures of Prosocial Development and Empathy

	Prosocial behavior teacher	Prosocial moral reasoning	Liked most	Helping most
Prosocial moral reasoning	.25*			
Liked most	.23*	.21*		
Helping most	.39*	.03	.38*	
Empathy	.16	.18*	.17*	.10

*$p < 0.05$

prosocial reasoning; children who were seen as prosocial by their teacher and were most liked by their classmates, used less hedonistic and more altruistic reasons for helping others in need.

Our third question concerned relations between perceived child rearing on the one hand and empathy and prosocial development on the other hand. These relations are presented in Table 4 (mothers) and Table 5 (fathers). Maternal support was positively related to prosocial

Table 4   *Relations Between Perceived Mother's Child rearing and Prosocial Development and Empathy*

	Support	Induction	Power assertion	Deman– dingness
Prosocial behavior according to teacher	.27*	−.05	−.05	.03
Prosocial moral reasoning	.22*	.18*	−.26*	.18*
Liked most	.04	.22*	−.21*	.19*
Helping most	−.05	.07	−.04	.09
Empathy	.12	.22*	−.28*	.34*

*p < 0.05

Table 5   *Relations Between Perceived Father's Child rearing and Prosocial Development and Empathy*

	Support	Induction	Power assertion	Deman– dingness
Prosocial behavior according to teacher	.05	−.11	−.02	.03
Prosocial moral reasoning	.05	.04	−.07	.17*
Liked most	.01	.26*	−.22*	.07
Helping most	−.06	.13	−.06	.00
Empathy	.04	.31*	−.21*	.23*

*p < 0.05

behavior in the classroom based on the teacher's reports and the
children's prosocial reasoning. Empathy was not related to perceived
maternal support. On the other hand, empathy was positively related
to induction and to demandingness and negatively to power assertion. Induction correlated positively with prosocial reasoning and
with being most liked by classmates. A similar pattern held for
demandingness. Demandingness was positively related to prosocial
reasoning and being most liked by classmates. Power assertion correlated negatively with prosocial reasoning and with being most liked
by classmates. From Table 4 we concluded that the child's empathy,
prosocial reasoning and popularity among classmates were positively
related to an inductive, demanding pattern of maternal child rearing
and negatively to maternal power assertion.

From Table 5 it was evident that perceived paternal induction and
demandingness were also positively related to empathy. Induction
also correlated positively with being most liked and demandingness
with prosocial reasoning. Paternal support was not related to empathy
or any measure of prosocial development. Paternal power assertion
was negatively related to empathy and being most liked by classmates.

In summary, we found significant relations between induction and
demandingness on the one hand and prosocial reasoning, empathy
and being most liked by classmates on the other. Power assertion,
however, was negatively associated with empathy, prosocial reasoning and being most liked by classmates. It was striking that the
school-related measures of prosocial behavior (measured by teacher
and classmates) were not related to child rearing.

From the data we concluded that power assertion, induction and
demandingness were related concepts and had to be studied simultaneously with regard to their effect on empathy and prosocial development. LISREL provides the opportunity to do so. For the LISREL-
analysis we constructed two latent child rearing factors; the first
consisting only of the variable support, the second with positive
loadings of induction and demandingness and a negative loading of
power assertion. From Table 1 and Table 2 we concluded that power
assertion, induction, and demandingness were highly correlated with
one another. Therefore, we decided to construct a latent factor with
estimated loadings of these three child-rearing measures. Support was
also related to these three measures, but the common variance was too
low to expect that support should have a substantive loading on that
latent factor. For that reason we constructed a second latent child-

rearing factor Support. In Table 6 (mothers) and Table 7 (fathers) the loadings of these variables on the two latent child-rearing factors are presented.

From Table 4 and Table 5 we concluded that empathy was positively related to induction and demandingness and negatively to power assertion. Therefore, we hypothesized that especially the latent factor with loadings of induction, demandingness and power assertion has a positive effect on a latent empathy-factor consisting of scores on the Bryant empathy scale. In the introduction we suggested an influence of support on empathy, but the results of Table 4 and Table 5 (no correlations between support and empathy) did not justify a hypothesized direct effect of support on empathy.

Because the correlations between the indices of prosocial behavior were high (see Table 3), we constructed only one latent factor for this construct consisting of the four measures of prosocial development: liked most, helping most, prosocial according to the teacher and quality of prosocial moral reasoning. The loadings of these four measured variables on the latent factor Prosocial development are presented in Table 6 and Table 7. From the results presented in Table 3, we hypothesized that empathy has a positive influence on the child's prosocial development. In summary, we tested the following model (see Figure 3) seperately for mothers and fathers:

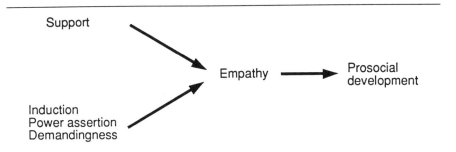

Figure 3   LISREL-model: Hypothesized relations between child rearing practices, empathy and prosocial development

The results of the LISREL-analyses are presented in Figure 4 (mothers) and Figure 5 (fathers). The strength of relationships between latent factors is represented by the standardized regression coefficients, along the arrows in Figure 4 and Figure 5. All hypothesized factor loadings and all regression-coefficients were statistically significant (alpha = .05). Also the overall-fit of the models was satisfactory

Table 6   Latent Factors in LISREL–analysis (Mothers) and Loadings of
           Measured Variables

		Latent factors		
	Support	Induction Power assertion Demandingness	Empathy	Prosocial development
Measured variables				
Support	1.00			
Induction		.67		
Power assertion		−.77		
Demandingness		.66		
Empathy			1.00	
Prosocial behavior according to teacher				.67
Prosocial reasoning				.34
Most liked				.48
Most helping				.54

Table 7   Latent Factors in LISREL–analysis (Fathers) and Loadings of
           Measured Variables

		Latent factors		
	Support	Induction Power assertion Demandingness	Empathy	Prosocial development
Measured variables				
Support	1.00			
Induction		.54		
Power assertion		−1.00		
Demandingness		.57		
Empathy			1.00	
Prosocial behavior according to teacher				.58
Prosocial reasoning				.28
Most liked				.54
Most helping				.62

(see the values for chi-square in Figure 4 and Figure 5). The goodness-of-fit (GFI) and the adjusted goodness-of-fit (AGFI) were .92 and .87 for mothers and .92 and .88 for fathers (see for criteria Lapsley & Quintana, 1989; Tanaka, 1987).

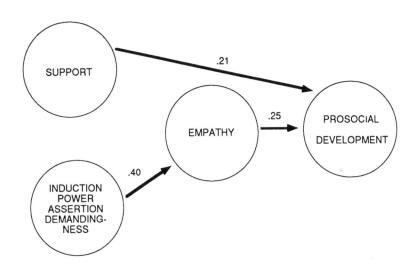

Figure 4   LISREL-model (mothers) (chi-square=37.07; df=26; p=0.074

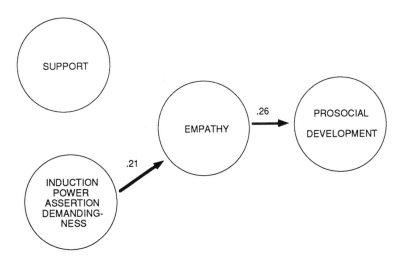

Figure 5   LISREL-model (fathers) (chi-square=38.45; df=28; p=0.090)

From the LISREL-analyses (Figure 4 and Figure 5) first, it appeared that maternal support had a moderate direct effect on the child's prosocial development. A second finding was that empathy had a positive influence on prosocial development. This influence was moderate, but statistically significant. Empathy was dependent on a child-rearing pattern that was characterized by induction and demandingness, in which parents used little power assertion. From these findings we concluded that empathy mediated between child rearing and prosocial development.

To control whether other models fitted better to the data, we tested two other models. In the first model empathy was not considered as an intervening, but as a dependent variable besides the dependent latent factor Prosocial development. That model did not fit as well as the models in Figure 4 and Figure 5 (chi-square = 40.83, d.f. = 27, p = .043, GFI = .92, AGFI = .86 for mothers and chi-square = 42.54, d.f. = 29, p = .050, GFI =.92, AGFI = .87 for fathers). A model in which empathy was not considered as a latent factor, but as an index of the latent factor "prosocial development", had even a poorer fit (chi-square = 51.70, d.f.= 26, p = .002, GFI = .90, AGFI = .83 for mothers and chi-square = 51.70, d.f.= 27, p = .003, GFI = .89, AGFI = .82 for fathers).

Discussion

From our research it became clear that demandingness and induction were positively related to each other and that both had a negative relation with power assertion. In the LISREL-analysis these three childrearing practices loaded on one latent factor. For this combined child-rearing factor, the label Authoritative may be appropriate; not in the sense Maccoby and Martin (1983) had given to this term, but in that of Baumrind (1971). In Maccoby and Martin's model authoritative child rearing is characterized by demandingness and responsiveness. In our study, however, support was relatively independent of the authoritative factor. Baumrind did not imply responsiveness as a main aspect of authoritative parenting. In her definition, authoritative child rearing means that parents appeal to their child's responsibility, make demands about mature behavior, and control whether their child behaves according to their expectations and demands. From our findings, we concluded that demanding parents were more inductive than power assertive when controlling. We may describe an authoritative parent as a parent who is demanding and inductive and someone who uses little power assertion. On the other hand, we may describe an authoritarian parent as a parent who is power assertive, not inductive and little demanding. The authoritarian parent restricts the child's behavior, does not accept deviations, nor gives responsibility to the child. The emphasis is more on the child's wrongdoing, whereas the authoritative parent is more concerned about the child's mature behavior.

The relations between child rearing on the one hand and empathy and prosocial development on the other hand were evident. An authoritative pattern of child rearing had a positive influence on the child's empathy and prosocial development. Moreover, in this study Eisenberg and Miller's conclusion about a moderate, but significant relation between empathy and prosocial behavior was confirmed. Empathy was positively related to two measures of prosocial development: prosocial reasoning and being most liked by classmates. No relations were found between empathy and prosocial behavior in the classroom as reported by teachers and classmates.

As we said before, the authoritative versus authoritarian dimension was relatively independent of the support-dimension. Moreover, only maternal support was related to prosocial development. This relation, however, was not mediated by empathy. Of course, there are other potential mediating links such as modeling effects, reinforcements, attributions, socio-cognitive conflicts and information-processing that could be triggered by parental behaviors. In regard to the influence of support, an explanation in terms of social learning is possible. Maybe the supportive mother is a model for her child to behave prosocially. The correlation between support and prosocial development was not very high. This may be due to the small variance in the variable of support. In our research a parent could give a supportive reaction in only two situations. In these two stories the child transgressed a norm or rule after he or she was provoked by others or while he or she was distressed. Because of the small variance, correlations between support and other variables could not become substantive.

Another important result of our study was the moderate, but significant relation between prosocial reasoning and prosocial behavior. In the literature, hardly any results can be found about this relation. Also the indices of prosocial behavior were related with one another. Children who were prosocial according to their teacher were also seen as such by their classmates. There was, however, one measure ("who helps most?") that was not related to empathy nor to child rearing. We suggest the following explanation. When we asked children to identify three children in their class who helped most, they had children in mind who helped with reading or arithmetic or some other academic task. They mentioned clever, not prosocial children in the class. However, when we asked peers to mention three children they liked most, they may have had other characteristics in mind. For instance, they may have refered to children who comforted other children, who were nice or fair, or who shared with other children. It is our opinion that report of the three most liked children is a better indicator for prosocial behavior than the children's nominations of three children who help in the class.

A final comment pertains to the way we measured child-rearing practices. We measured parental behavior as perceived by the child. That does not mean that this parental behavior is the same as their actual behavior. Nevertheless, our findings underscore the importance of using the child's perceptions and reports of parental child-rearing practices, particularly when the relations between child rearing and the child's prosocial development are studied.

References

Baumrind, D. (1971). Current patterns of parental authority. *Development psychology Monograph, 4*.

Bryant, B. (1982). An index of empathy for children and adolescents. *Child Development, 53*, 413-425.

Coopersmith, S. (1967). *The antecedents of self-esteem*. San Francisco: Freeman.

Eisenberg-Berg, N. (1979). Development of children's prosocial moral judgment. *Developmental Psychology, 15*, 128-137.

Eisenberg-Berg, N., & Hand, M. (1979). The relationship of preschools' reasoning about prosocial moral conflicts to prosocial behavior. *Child Development, 15*, 128-137.

Eisenberg, N., Lennon, R., & Roth, K. (1983). Prosocial development: a longitudinal study. *Developmental Psychology, 19*, 846-855.

Eisenberg, N., & Miller, P. A. (1987). The relation of empathy to prosocial and related behaviors. *Psychological Bulletin, 101*, 91-119.

Hoffman, M. L. (1963). Parent discipline and the child's consideration for others. *Child Development, 34*, 573-588.

Hoffman, M. L. (1970). Moral development. In H.P. Mussen (Ed.), *Carmichael's Handbook of Child Psychology*. New York: Wiley.

Hoffman, M. L. (1975). Altruistic behavior and the parent-child relationship. *Journal of Personality and Social Psychology, 11*, 937-943.

Hoffman, M. L. (1976). Empathy, roletaking, guilt and development of altruistic motives. In Th. Lickona (Ed.), *Moral development and moral behavior*, New York: Rinehart & Winston.

Hoffman, M. L. (1982). Development of prosocial motivation; empathy and guilt. In N. Eisenberg (Ed.), *The development of prosocial behavior*. New York: Academic Press.

Hoffman, M. L., & Saltzstein, H. D. (1967). Parent discipline and the child's moral development. *Journal of Personality and Social Psychology, 5*, 45-57.

Lapsley, D. K., & Quintana, S. M. (1989). Mental capacity and role taking; a structural equations approach. *Merrill Palmer Quarterly, 35*, 143-163.

Maccoby, E. E. (1980). *Social development*. San Diego: Harcourt Brace Jovanovitch.

Maccoby, E. E., & J. A. Martin (1983). Socialization in the context of the family: parent-child interaction. In P. H. Mussen (Ed.), *Handbook of Child Psychology. Vol. IV. Socialization, personality and social development*. New York: Wiley.

Magnusson, D. K., & V. L. Allen (1983). An interactional perspective for human development. In: D. Magnusson and V. L. Allen (Eds.), *Human development: An interactional perspective*. New York: Academic Press.

Radke-Yarrow, M., Zahn-Waxler, C., & Chapman, M. (1983). Children's prosocial dispositions and behavior. In P. H. Mussen (Ed.), *Handbook of child psychology, Vol.4*. New York: Wiley.

Rollins, B. C., & D. L. Thomas (1979). Parental support, power and control techniques in the socialization of children. In W. R. Burr, R. Hill, F. I. Nye, & I. L. Reiss (Eds.), *Contemporary theories about the family. Vol. 1*. London: Free Press.

Staub, E. (1979). *Positive social behavior and morality Vol. 2*. New York: Academic Press.

Tanaka, J. S. (1987). "How big is big enough?", Sample size and goodness of fit in structural equation models with latent variables. *Child Development, 56*, 134-146.

Weir, K., & G. Duveen (1981). Further development and validation of the Prosocial Behaviour Questionnaire for use by teachers. *Journal of child psychology and psychiatry, 22*, 357-374.

R.J. Iannotti, E.M. Cummings, B. Pierrehumbert,
M.J. Milano, C. Zahn-Waxler

Parental Influences on Prosocial Behavior and Empathy in Early Childhood

There can be little doubt that young children, before the age of three, demonstrate complex social behaviors including prosocial behavior (Dunn & Kendrick, 1979; Hay, 1979; Radke-Yarrow, Zahn-Waxler & Chapman, 1983; Rheingold, Hay & West, 1976), evidence of early perspective taking (Lempers, Flavell & Flavell, 1977; Liben, 1978; Zahn-Waxler, Radke-Yarrow & Brady-Smith, 1977), and empathy (Halperin & Iannotti, 1989; Hoffman & Levine, 1976). Most of this research has been cross-sectional, raising questions as to whether these early manifestations of social cognition and prosocial behavior are stable, whether these are early precursors for later prosocial acts, and whether facilitation of prosocial behaviors in the early years has consequences for later childhood.

Stability of prosocial behavior across settings or over short periods of time is generally in the low range, with correlations between different measures of prosocial behaviors of approximately .30 being most representative (e.g., Eisenberg-Berg & Hand, 1979; Hay, 1979; Rushton, 1976; Underwood & Moore, 1982; Yarrow & Waxler, 1976). Studies which rely on composite measures report somewhat higher correlations (see review by Radke-Yarrow et al., 1983). Unfortunately, there are few longitudinal studies of prosocial behaviors, particularly that examine prosocial behavior of toddlers as predictors of prosocial behavior in early childhood (see review by Mussen & Eisenberg-Berg, 1977). In the present study, observational categories of prosocial behavior were combined to investigate developmental changes from two to five years of age.

The presence or absence of stability in prosocial behavior has theoretical implications. Stability may exist in the internalization of societal norms or expectations, in the individual characteristics which mediate prosocial responses such as social, cognitive and affective processes, or in the socialization processes or social situations which facilitate prosocial behavior such as parental child-rearing patterns. Each of these processes may be evident in early childhood. The mediational role of social-cognitive processes and influence of parental beliefs and behaviors are examined in the current study.

Empathy, the ability to understand and share the inner affective state of another person, has been suggested as one example of a social-cognitive mediator of prosocial behavior, certainly for older children and perhaps for young children as well (Feshbach, 1975; Hoffman, 1975; Iannotti, 1975; Shantz, 1975). Definitions of empathy may differ as do the methods for operationalizing the construct. The empathic response may be differentially influenced by situational cues versus characteristics of the other's emotional response (Deutsch & Madle, 1975; Iannotti, 1975, 1985). Reliance on situational cues may reflect the application of social-cognitive processes toward understanding the emotional situation (Gove & Keating, 1979; Iannotti, 1975) and appears to increase with age (Iannotti, 1977). The current study operationalizes empathy so as to differentiate response to situational and affective cues. The relationship between empathy and altruism is dependent on the age of the child, the measures of empathy and altruism, and the context for measuring both (Eisenberg & Lennon, 1983; Eisenberg, McCreath & Ahn, 1988; Radke-Yarrow et al., 1983). There has been relatively little research examining longitudinal relationships between prosocial behavior and empathy, particularly whether early sociocognitive behaviors relate to later empathic processes.

One focus for theoretical discussion of the development of prosocial behaviors and empathy has been the role of perspective-taking skills as precursors to and necessary components of a genuine altruistic or empathic response. Measures of perspective taking have been positively correlated with helping and sharing, and attempts to enhance perspective-taking skills have produced increased prosocial behavior (Ahammer & Murray, 1979; Buckley, Siegel & Ness, 1979; Iannotti, 1978; Staub, 1971). Perspective-taking ability may influence the dynamics of parent-child interaction and parental expectations for prosocial behavior in their young children (Stewart & Marvin, 1984) and may affect the dynamics of peer interactions as well (LeMare &

Rubin, 1987). Early forms of perspective taking and their relationship to current and subsequent prosocial and empathic behaviors are examined in the current study.

The dynamics of the parent-child relationship and the socialization practices of the parent may have a direct effect on prosocial behavior or may have an indirect effect through these mediating processes. An adjunct of this question is whether early socialization practices relate to the later development and expression of the empathic response. Parental use of reasoning or reasoned guidance have been related to the development of empathy (Abraham, Kuehl & Chrisopherson, 1983; Jensen, Peery, Adams & Gaynard, 1981). Recognition and expression of affect are often considered to be essential elements in the development of empathy (Hoffman, 1975). It is not surprising then that parental warmth, intimacy, and freedom of expression have been related to empathy in children (Abraham et al., 1983; Feshbach, 1978). Mothers who explain distress and provide empathic caregiving also promote prosocial behavior in their young children (Zahn-Waxler, Radke-Yarrow & King, 1979). Looking at the process from another perspective, Janssens, Gerris, and Janssen (1989) found that empathy in children may mediate the effect of child-rearing practices on prosocial behavior in children. The current study examines the relationship of early parent-child interactions and early prosocial behaviors with later empathic responses.

The influence of parents on prosocial behavior may be direct. In addition to parental modeling, parental warmth, and nurturance (Baumrind, 1971; Bryant & Crockenberg, 1980; Feshbach, 1978; Rutherford & Mussen, 1968; Yarrow, Scott & Waxler, 1973), parental techniques including use of power assertion, induction, and cognitive techniques (Dlugokinski & Firestone, 1974; Hoffman & Saltzstein, 1967; Perry, Bussey, & Feiberg, 1981), and encouragement of prosocial acts (Biron, Ramos & Higa, 1977) have all been identified as having positive or negative relations to the subsequent development of altruism. Grusec and Dix (1986) emphasize the importance of internalization and generalization in the development of prosocial behavior and suggest that parental modeling with firm demands for appropriate behavior accompanied by reasons fosters these processes. The quality of the parent-child relationship may also be reflected in the attachment relationship. Security of attachment has been shown to have both long- and short-term consequences for social and prosocial interactions with adults and peers (La Freniere, 1983; Londerville & Main, 1981; Pastor, 1981).

It is expected that parents of toddlers who model prosocial behavior, exhibit perspective taking, explicitly encourage prosocial behavior, show warmth and nurturance, use induction or reasoning, or permit independence or choice have children with increased levels of prosocial behavior or empathy at two and at five years of age. Parents who use authoritarian control, use punishment without age-appropriate rationales, or who have not established a secure attachment relationship are expected to have children with lower levels of prosocial behavior and empathy.

Research Questions
The research questions which are addressed in this study are:
1. What are the determinants of social and prosocial behaviors in early childhood?
2. Are social and prosocial behaviors stable during these early years?
3. Are maternal attitudes and behaviors stable during these early years?
4. Do social-cognitive processes influence early social and prosocial behaviors?
5. Do maternal attitudes and behaviors predict children's social and prosocial behaviors?

Methods

Subjects
Mothers and their two-year-old children (mean = 2.4, S.D. = 0.3) participated in three play sessions, each session involving two mothers and two children. Twenty-six mothers were asked to invite a child, who was a familiar playmate, and his/her mother to the first session. Two months after the first session, these 52 mother-child pairs returned with a new familiar mother and peer (different in gender from the peer previously seen) for a second session. Three months later, they returned with the first familiar peer and mother for a third session. A home visit followed this third session in which each mother completed additional measures. Forty-nine mother-child pairs participated in all three sessions and the home visit: 28 males, 21 females; predominantly middle class (Hollingshead, 1975), intact families (mean = 51, S.D. = 13). When these children were approximately five years old (mean = 5.0, S.D. = 0.4) 43 of these mother-child pairs returned for a fourth visit with a new same-sex, familiar peer

and the peer's mother. Thirty-nine mothers completed additional measures at home and returned them by mail. Analyses were performed on the 43 mother-child pairs (19 females, 24 males) who participated in all four laboratory sessions and separate analyses were performed for the 39 mothers completing all measures. The analyses reported here were part of a broader study that also examined children's responses to adult conflict and parental depression. These variables had no significant effects on the measures reported in the current study.

Procedures at Two Years of Age
Each session lasted 35 min and was videotaped through two one-way mirrors at opposite ends of the room. After a brief introduction and discussion of the procedures, two toddlers and their mothers were escorted to a fully furnished efficiency apartment. A standard set of age-appropriate toys was located on the floor in the center of the room. During the first two sessions mothers were given paper and pencil tasks and instructed not to initiate interactions with the children or to interrupt children's interactions unless something occurred which made them uncomfortable or they felt was dangerous. If the children initiated contact, mothers were instructed to respond in a normal manner. Two adult researchers entered the room at five minute intervals according to a set script. These adults simulated different emotional interactions but did not interact directly with the children except to offer a beverage toward the end of the session (for a complete description of the procedure see Cummings, Iannotti & Zahn-Waxler, 1985). These simulations had no effect on the social responsivity or prosocial behaviors of the children. Each child's social responsivity and prosocial behavior to a child or adult during these sessions were coded. Attachment was coded at the end of each session by evaluating the child's response to separation from and reunion with his or her mother.

In the third session mothers were encouraged to interact with the children as they normally would. Because the children were familiar friends, mothers were also quite friendly and these sessions were marked by considerable socializing between mothers as well as interactions between mothers and children. This session included play periods guided by each mother to assure a more than adequate sample of mother-child interactions. Mother's child-rearing and perspective-taking behaviors were coded from this session as well as the child's social responsivity.

During a subsequent home visit mothers completed several additional questionnaires including the Child-Rearing Practices Report Q-Sort (Block, 1965).

Indices at Two Years of Age
Measure of Social Responsivity. The index of *responsiveness* was designed to evaluate the extent to which one participant responded to the social initiatives of another (see Pierrehumbert, Iannotti, Cummings & Zahn-Waxler, 1989, for a complete description of the coding system). The index was not designed to assess the frequency of social interactions, but rather the tendency to respond, given an opportunity to respond.

The interactions were coded by two observers. Interobserver agreement at two and five was 94 percent. Responsivity could only be computed when the subject had opportunities to respond, i.e., when he or she was the target of partner's initiatives—mother or peer. Therefore, at each age level all sessions were used to compute the index.

Prosocial Behavior. Prosocial behavior was coded for the first two sessions, a total of 70 min. Prosocial behaviors were defined as acts of sharing, helping, cooperating or compassion initiated by the target child toward the peer or another adult in the room, usually the child's mother. Sharing was defined as giving, exchanging or offering an object to another individual. Helping was defined as performing a task or giving information which assists another person. Cooperation was defined as taking turns with an object of which neither participant had possession or working together to complete something which would have been more difficult to complete alone. There had to be mutual involvement and repetition or alternating turns for an act to be coded as cooperation. Compassion was defined as an act of affection following distress in the other person. Distress behaviors included crying, whimpering, and verbal, facial, or other expressions of distress or upset. Acts of affection included verbal expressions of affection and physical acts such as hugging, kissing, or patting. Observer agreement for identifying a prosocial act was 94 percent and agreement for the different categories of prosocial behavior once a prosocial act was identified was 100 percent.

Attachment. Quality of attachment to the mother was assessed from the child's responses to separation from and reunion with his/her mother using the criteria of Ainsworth, Blehar, Waters and Wall (1978) for secure and insecure (ambivalent or avoidant) attachment. Although these criteria were originally developed for the entire Ainsworth procedure, the reunion episode was the primary focus. In this variant of Ainsworth's procedure, first the mother of the peer, then the target mother, left the two children alone after approximately 28 min of peer interaction, saying "I'll be back." Mothers observed the session through the one-way mirror and returned together if there was extreme distress. All mothers returned after one minute. "Secure" (B) toddlers were identified as those who actively sought contact or interaction with the mother during reunion and were effectively quieted by contact with the mother. "Insecure-resistant" (C) toddlers were difficult to comfort during reunion and mixed contact seeking with pushing away. "Insecure-avoidant" (A) toddlers ignored and/or avoided the mother during reunion. The original procedure was designed for twelve month olds; these categories for the reunion behavior have been shown to be valid through two years of age (Lamb, Thompson, Gardner & Charnov, 1985). Interobserver agreement for attachment classification was 92 percent. Coders were blind with regard to other categories of coding and only observed the separation procedure.

Perspective Taking Tasks. Following the third session, measures of perspective taking were administered using the child's mother as the source of information or as the target for many of the tasks. The tasks were: a) Language. In an adaptation of a procedure used by Bretherton and Beeghly (1982), each mother was asked to give examples of her child's use of eight "external" words which were observable manifestations of potentially internal processes, e.g., hug, sleep, eat, and laugh, and eight "internal" words which referred to internal states or processes, e.g., love, tired, hungry, and happy. A score was derived to reflect the child's recognition that others experience internal states or processes. b) Hiding and Showing. These tasks, adapted from Lempers et al. (1977), required that children consider their mothers' spatial perspective in order to hide objects, e.g., blocks, hands, or self, from her or show objects, e.g., pictures, only the hands, or back, to her. c) Penny-Hiding. The Devries Penny Hiding Task (1970) was scored to indicate whether the child had a strategy for guessing the location of the hidden object, a strategy for hiding the object, and the effectiveness of hiding the objects. Scores from each task were standardized and then summed to derive a total perspective-taking score (scoring procedures for each task can be obtained from the first author). Reliability of the perspective-taking tasks was .73.

Observational Coding of Mother's Behaviors. Mother-child interactions during the third session were coded for mother's child-rearing behaviors and mother's display of perspective taking with her child. Reliabilities ranged from .75 to 1.00 and averaged .88. Four subscales were identified as of theoretical interest for influencing prosocial behavior or social cognitions in the children. Mother's interactions with her child which were judged to *promote prosocial behaviors* included verbal statements which encourage prosocial behavior, e.g., "It's her turn," and modeling prosocial behavior by sharing, helping, cooperating, or showing compassion to the other child, other adult, or her own child. *Encourage perspective taking* was coded when a mother: a) Directed her child's attention to the feelings of others in room, e.g., "Why is John so sad?"; b) Directed her child's attention to his/her own feelings, e.g., "You're happy because you get to ride the horse now."; c) Directed her child's attention to another's thoughts, e.g., "I don't know what you want."; d) Directed her child's attention to his/ her own thoughts, e.g., "You thought that was the big block."; or e) Used another person as point of reference, e.g., "It's the one in front of Paul."

Mother's attempts to control or direct the behavior of her child were also identified. Categories of interest include: *soft control*, when the mother qualified commands and/or used questions to direct the child's behavior, e.g., Would you like to..., Why don't you..., How about if we..., Maybe you could..., and bargains or bribes, e.g., "You can have juice if you finish cleaning."; and maternal *warmth*, coded when mothers made affectionate statements, e.g., "You're mommy's friend, sweetie."; made positive statements about the child's behavior, "That's great!"; or displayed affection in expression or behavior, e.g., smiled with eye contact; held or hugged her child.

Mother's display of perspective taking with her child was coded as an indication of the mother's use of perspective taking skills in social situations and as a potential influence on her child's perspective taking as a model. The behaviors during Session 3 which reflected perspective taking skills included when the mother: a) Simplified or provided more information when her child did not respond or did not understand; b) Showed sensitivity to her child's visual perspective, e.g., moved objects into or out of her child's field of vision or gave location information relative to the child's visual perspective; c) Demonstrated an awareness of her child's wants, thoughts, or feelings without her child explicitly expressing these, e.g., after child stared at play horse, mother says, "The horse'll be yours in just a little while."

During a subsequent home visit mothers completed the Child-Rearing Practices Report Q-Sort (Block, 1965). The six subscales of interest were *expression of affect* (e.g., "I express affection by hugging, kissing, and holding my child."), *encourage independence* (e.g., "I teach my child that s/he is responsible for what happens to him/her."), *rational guidance*, (e.g., "I talk it over and reason with my child when he/she misbehaves."), *anxiety induction* (e.g., "I teach my child that in one way or another punishment will find them when s/he is bad."), *non-punitive punishment* (e.g., "I punish my child by taking away a privilege he or she otherwise would have had."), and *authoritarian control* (e.g., "Physical punishment is the best form of discipline" and "I have strict, well-established rules.").

Procedures at Five Years of Age
Forty-three of the original mother-child pairs returned with a new familiar peer for a *follow-up session* at five years of age, which was similar to the first two sessions in structure. In the first 30 minutes mothers were given paper and pencil tasks and similar instructions not to interact with the children unless approached. In the last 5 min of the 35 min session the paper and pencil tasks were collected and mothers were reminded that they were free to interact with each other and the children in a normal manner.

Children's behaviors were coded for *prosocial behavior* with codes similar to those at two years of age. Verbal initiations for prosocial behavior, which were not coded at two due to the lack of comprehensible verbal statements by the two-year-olds, were added at five years of age. Observer agreement for individual categories of prosocial behavior at age five ranged from 69 to 100 percent, and agreement for the total prosocial behavior score was 90 percent.

The *social responsiveness* coding was repeated for a subsample of 33 five-year-old children. To avoid possible effects of other activities during the session and to balance the time periods when mothers were available to interact with those when mothers were busy completing forms, responsiveness was coded during two episodes of the follow-up session: a) The first five min free-play episode, and b) The five min free-play episode in which the mothers were free to interact were coded.

Empathy. Several individual measures were administered following the session including a measure of empathy. The measure of empathy (Iannotti, 1978, 1985) differentiated responses to affective and situational cues. Sixteen photographs depicting consistent and inconsistent situational and emotional cues were used to assess the children's own affective response and their understanding of another's feelings. Responses were scored to determine whether the children were more likely to respond to situational or emotional cues when indicating their emotional response to the stimuli. Credit was given for *emotional matching* when the child's self-report of his/her emotions matched the situational and affective cues of one of the 8 stimuli with matching (congruent) situational and affective cues. *Affective empathy* was scored when the child's self-report of his/her emotions matched the affective cues of one of the 8 stimuli with non-matching (incongruent) situational and affective cues. If the child's self-report of his/her emotions matched the situational cues of one of these 8 stimuli with non-matching (incongruent) situational and affective cues it was scored as *situational empathy*. The score for each of these categories of empathy could range from 0 to 8.

The Child-Rearing Practices Report Q-Sort was administered again to the mothers after the session at five years.

Results

The means and standard deviations of all measures are displayed in Tables 1 and 2 for mothers and children respectively. The high frequency of most child-rearing behaviors reflects the design of the third session which promoted mother-child interaction. There were no significant gender differences for any of the measures of children's behaviors and negligible differences in mothers' child-rearing attitudes and behaviors. All subsequent analyses were collapsed across gender.

Changes in behavior from when the children were two years old to the session at five years of age were examined for mother's child-rearing attitudes, social responsiveness, and prosocial behavior to peers, the only measures which were comparable at both ages. There were significant age effects for responsiveness to peers, $t(32) = 7.42$, $p < .001$, responsiveness to mothers, $t(32) = 6.31$, $p < .001$, and prosocial behaviors to peers, $t(42) = 2.11$, $p < .05$, all indicating increased social and prosocial behavior at five years of age.

A series of correlational analyses were performed in order to examine relations among measures at each age level and between measures across age levels.

Table 1   Means (and Standard Deviations) of Mother's Behaviors for
          Children at 2 and 5 Years of Age

Behavior	Girls		Boys	
Mother's Child-Rearing Behaviors for Two-Year-Old Children				
Promote Prosocial Behaviors	5.7	(4.78)	8.4	(6.14)
Encourage Perspective Taking	24.7	(15.49)	24.9	(16.00)
Soft Control	53.2	(22.46)	43.8	(16.64)
Warmth	49.7	(23.63)	41.9	(20.74)
Mother's Display of Perspective Taking	51.2	(34.73)	39.4	(31.61)
Mother's Child-Rearing Attitudes for Two-Year-Old Children				
Expression of Affect**	6.5	(.41)	6.2	(.41)
Encourage Independence	4.7	(.66)	4.9	(.94)
Rational Guidance	6.2	(.39)	6.2	(.53)
Anxiety Induction	2.8	(1.35)	3.0	(1.11)
Non-Punitive Punishment	4.7	(.66)	4.9	(.94)
Authoritarian Control	2.4	(.35)	2.5	(.54)
Mother's Child-Rearing Attitudes for Five-Year-Old Children				
Expression of Affect	6.3	(.46)	6.1	(.45)
Encourage Independence	4.6	(.57)	4.9	(.62)
Rational Guidance	6.2	(.53)	5.9	(.89)
Anxiety Induction*	2.1	(.99)	3.0	(1.19)
Non-Punitive Punishment	5.0	(1.17)	4.8	(1.02)
Authoritarian Control	2.2	(.32)	2.5	(.53)

Note: Means for Mother's Child-Rearing Behaviors are frequency during a
      35 min session.

**$p < .01$ for gender differences in means.
*$p < .05$ for gender differences in means.

Table 2   Means (and Standard Deviations) of Children's Behaviors at 2
and 5 Years of Age

Behavior	Girls		Boys	
Child Behaviors at 2 Years of Age				
Social Responsiveness to Peers	1.35	(.31)	1.36	(.42)
Social Responsiveness to Mother	1.40	(.31)	1.48	(.37)
Prosocial Behaviors to Peers	3.7	(2.10)	3.1	(2.05)
Prosocial Behaviors to Adults	1.7	(1.44)	1.5	(1.60)
Early Forms of Perspective Taking	0.32	(7.61)	-0.34	(5.46)
Child Behaviors at 5 Years of Age				
Social Responsiveness to Peers	2.52	(1.01)	2.71	(1.04)
Social Responsiveness to Mother	1.88	(.56)	2.04	(.39)
Prosocial Behaviors to Peers	5.7	(5.02)	4.5	(3.60)
Emotional Matching	5.0	(2.11)	3.9	(2.15)
Affective Empathy	2.7	(1.80)	2.8	(2.13)
Situational Empathy	2.7	(1.98)	2.8	(1.92)

Note: Mean for child's prosocial behavior is frequency during 35 min
session.

Correlations Among Measures at Two Years of Age
Relations between mother's self reports and observed behaviors. The correlations between mother's self-reported child-rearing practices when
her child was two and observed interactions with her two year old are
shown in Table 3. As can be seen in the patterns of these correlations,
mother's reports of child-rearing beliefs which encourage independence and the use of rational guidance were generally positively
related to the observed behaviors which were expected to promote
prosocial behavior and the development of social skills. Mother's self
reports of anxiety induction, non-punitive punishment, and authoritarian control were generally negatively related to the observed
behaviors, with only negative correlations reaching statistical signifi-

cance. Promoting prosocial behavior and warmth were positively related to self-reports of encouraging independence, $r(41) = .32$, $p < .05$, and $r(41) = .41$, $p < .01$, respectively, and negatively correlated with anxiety induction, $r(41) = -.30$, $p < .05$, and $r(41) = -.31$, $p < .05$, respectively. Soft control was negatively correlated with mother's reports of non-punitive punishment, $r(41) = -.32$, $p < .05$.

Table 3   Correlations Between Mother's Observed Behaviors at Age 2 and Mother's Self-Report at 2 and 5

| | Mother's Observed Behaviors for Two-Year-Old Children | | | | |
Self-Report at 2	Promoting Prosocial	Encouraging Perspectives	Soft Control	Warmth	Perspective Taking
Expression of Affect	.11	.04	.22	.13	-.07
Encourage Independence	.32*	.29a	.29a	.41**	.28a
Rational Guidance	.03	.28a	.29a	.07	.09
Anxiety Induction	-.30*	-.26a	-.18	-.31*	-.08
Non-Punitive Punishment	-.09	.07	-.32*	-.18	-.24
Authoritarian Control	-.20	-.29a	-.15	-.10	.14

| | Mother's Observed Behaviors for Two-Year-Old Children | | | | |
Self-Report at 5	Promoting Prosocial	Encouraging Perspectives	Soft Control	Warmth	Perspective Taking
Expression of Affect	.02	.08	.06	-.01	-.01
Encourage Independence	.05	.00	.23	.34*	.41*
Rational Guidance	-.03	.14	.39*	.02	.01
Anxiety Induction	-.21	-.23	-.26	-.35*	-.05
Non-Punitive Punishment	-.03	-.05	-.29a	.00	-.36*
Authoritarian Control	-.12	-.33a	-.15	-.29a	.07

Note: N = 43 at two year of age and 35 at five years of age; ap < .10
*p < .05, **p < .01.

Relations between mother's and child's behaviors. Children's responsiveness to peers was negatively related to mother's encouraging prosocial behavior, $r(41) = -.33$, $p < .05$, but responsiveness to mother was positively related to mother's encouraging perspective taking, $r(41) = .34$, $p < .05$, soft control, $r(41) = .42$, $p < .01$, and warmth (see Table 4). Children's prosocial behaviors to peer, $r(41) = .31$, $p < .05$, and

Table 4   Correlations Between Mother's Observed Behaviors and Child's Behaviors at Age Two and Five

| Child's Behaviors at Two | Mother's Observed Behaviors at Two | | | | |
	Promoting Prosocial	Encouraging Perspectives	Soft Control	Warmth	Perspective Taking
Responsive to Peers	-.33*	-.23	-.01	.06	-.00
Responsive to Mother -.04		.08	.34*	.42**	.30a
Prosocial to Peers	.31*	.20	-.02	-.03	-.28a
Prosocial to Adults	.50***	.33*	.13	.13	-.17
Perspective Taking Tasks	-.04	-.17	-.08	-.13	-.33*
Attachment	.25	-.05	.18	.05	.07

| Child's Behaviors at Five | Mother's Observed Behaviors at Five | | | | |
	Promoting Prosocial	Encouraging Perspectives	Soft Control	Warmth	Perspective Taking
Responsive to Peers	.06	-.34a	-.04	.36a	-.12
Responsive to Mother .18		.25	.52**	.46*	.21
Prosocial to Peers	.00	-.09	-.30a	-.10	-.22
Response to Empathy Stimuli					
Emotional Matching	-.17	-.05	.14	.14	.18
Affective Empathy	-.21	-.08	.13	-.04	.07
Situational Empathy	.17	.07	-.05	.03	.07

Note: At two year of age N = 43; At five years of age N = 30 for responsiveness, N=40 for prosocial behavior and empathy stimuli. ap < .10, *p < .05, **p < .01., ***p < .001

to mother, $r(41) = .50$, $p < .001$, were both positively related to encouraging prosocial behaviors by the mother. There were no significant relationships between the attachment relationship and mother's observed behaviors.

Mother's report of expression of affect was related to the child's prosocial behaviors to peers; $r(47) = .31$, $p < .05$; and to adults; $r(47) = .28$, $p < .10$ (not shown in Table 4). There were no significant relationships between the children's performance on the perspective taking tasks and their social or prosocial behaviors in the sessions.

Correlations Between Measures at Two and Five Years of Age.
Relations between mother's behaviors at two and child's behaviors at five.
Mother's self-reported child-rearing practices were generally stable from two to five: expression of affect, $r(37) = .21$; encourage independence, $r(37) = .54$, $p < .001$; rational guidance, $r(37) = .39$, $p < .05$; anxiety induction, $r(37) = .49$, $p < .01$; non-punitive punishment, $r(37) = .47$, $p < .01$; authoritarian control, $r(37) = .59$, $p < .001$. The relations between mother's observed behaviors with her two year old and her self-reported practices at five, shown in Table 3, has much the same pattern as the correlations at two. Significant correlations were positive for encouraging independence and rational guidance and negative for anxiety induction and non-punitive punishment.

Mother's social behaviors with her child at two were related to her child's social and prosocial behaviors at 5, but there were no significant correlations for the measures of the child's empathic behaviors (see Table 4). The strongest relationships continued to be between mother's behaviors at two and the child's interactions with the mother at five. The child's responsiveness to the mother was positively correlated with encouraging perspective taking, $r(28) = .52$, $p < .01$, and with soft control, $r(28) = .46$, $p < .05$. The child's peer interactions were not as clearly related to the mother's earlier interactions with the child.

Mother's self-reports at five for use of non-punitive control and expression of affect were positively related to prosocial behavior to peers at five (not shown in Table 4); $r(33) = .39$, $p < .05$, and $r(33) = .35$, $p < .05$, respectively; and anxiety induction was positively related to affective empathy, $r(33) = .39$, $p < .05$.

Relations between child's behaviors at two and five. There was no evident for stability of specific children's behaviors from two to five years of age, i.e., behaviors observed at two were not significantly correlated with the same behavior codes at five, but prosocial behavior at two was significantly correlated with verbal prosocial statements at five, $r(41) = .31, p < .05$. There was other evidence that behaviors at two predicted behaviors at five across measures (see Table 5). The quality of the attachment relationship between mother and child at two predicted prosocial behavior toward peers at five, $r(41) = .30, p < .05$, and was a marginal predictor of responsiveness to mother at five, $r(31) = .30, p < .10$. Responsiveness to peers at two predicted emotional matching, $r(41) = .34, p < .05$, and affective empathy, $r(41) = .45, p < .01$. Perspective taking at two was marginally related to situational empathy, $r(41) = .29, p < .10$.

Table 5   Correlations Between Two-Year-Old Child's Behaviors in Sessions 1 and 2 and Child's Social, Prosocial, and Empathic Behaviors at Five Years

| Child's Behaviors at Five | Child's Behaviors at Two Years | | | | | |
	Responsive to Peers	Responsive to Mother	Prosocial to Peer	Prosocial to Adult	Perspective Taking	Attachment
Responsive to Peers	.06	-.05	.09	.13	.12	.17
Responsive to Mother	-.07	.25	-.05	.06	-.08	.30a
Prosocial to Peers	-.27a	.02	.22	.16	-.19	.30*
Response to Empathy Stimuli						
Emotional Matching	.34*	.07	-.11	-.21	.17	-.12
Affective Empathy	.45**	.01	-.06	-.14	-.26a	-.04
Situational Empathy	-.27a	-.08	-.07	.00	.29a	-.06

Note: N=33 for responsiveness, N=43 for prosocial behavior and empathy stimuli.
       ap < .10, *p < .05, **p < .01.

There were no significant correlations between empathy and responsiveness or total prosocial behavior, but situational empathy was significantly related to compassion at five years of age, $r(41) = .31$, $p < .05$.

Discussion

Early childhood is marked by increased social activity and development of social skills (Eckerman & Stein, 1982; Radke-Yarrow et al., 1983). The current longitudinal data provide further evidence of increased social behavior with peers during early childhood. Both social and prosocial behaviors toward peers increased from two to five years of age. Social responsiveness to mothers also increased during this period. The increased interaction with both mothers and peers suggests that the development of social relations with peers is not a replacement for contact with mothers but rather that children are expanding their social system while also becoming more responsive to the social initiatives of others.

While stability has previously been demonstrated during this period of rapid social development (Cummings, Iannotti & Zahn-Waxler, 1989), it is not evident in all social behaviors. There were no significant correlations between the child's prosocial behavior at two and at five. To the extent that stability exists it is more evident in the mother's child-rearing attitudes or perhaps in the relationship of the child with the mother. Five of the six child-rearing attitudes assessed in the mother when her child was two were related to her child-rearing attitudes when her child was five. The quality of the attachment between mother and child assessed at two years of age also predicted the responsiveness of the child to the mother at five.

In addition to the stability of child-rearing attitudes, there is evidence that the mother's child-rearing attitudes at two related to her interactions with her child at two, and that her interactions at two correlated with her child's social behaviors and with her own attitudes at five. The stability of the mother's social interactions with her child across this period was not examined. Encouraging independence appears to be the child-rearing attitude which is most clearly related to mother's social behaviors. Encouraging independence was significantly related to promoting prosocial behavior and warmth with trends indicating associations with encouraging perspective taking, using perspective taking in social interactions, and giving the child choices, or the appearance of choice, on issues of control. Encouraging independence may facilitate internalization of social norms and promote self-other differentiation, each important for the development of prosocial and perspective taking behaviors. The negative correlations of mother's social behaviors with child-rearing attitudes of non-punitive punishment and authoritarian control were consistent with expectations (Dlugokinski & Firestone, 1974; Hoffman & Saltzstein, 1967; Perry, Bussey, & Freiberg, 1981).

Similar patterns of relationships exist between mother's social behaviors at two and her child-rearing attitudes at five. Mother's positive social behaviors at two, specifically warmth and perspective taking, was still associated with encouraging independence at five. Soft control at two was correlated with rational guidance at five. Among the negative indicators, warmth at two was related to anxiety induction at five and perspective taking at two was related to non-punitive punishment. The results for mother's child-rearing attitudes and behaviors suggest that there is a relationship between attitudes and behaviors and that mother's child-rearing patterns have some stability during her child's early development. Stability may develop from the dynamic of the mother-child interaction or in the persistence of the mother's child-rearing patterns.

Given that stability may exist in the mother-child relationship, what features of a mother's social interactions with her child promote the development of social and prosocial behaviors? Mother's positive social behaviors appear to foster positive child-mother interactions more than child-peer interactions. For example, a mother promoting prosocial behavior of her child toward others was more likely to receive prosocial behavior from her child. Her child was also more likely to exhibit prosocial behavior toward peers but less likely to be responsive to peers. Children of mothers who exhibit warmth, encourage perspective taking, and use soft control techniques were more likely to be responsive to their mothers. When placed in a situation where both mother and peer are present, these children, while showing positive behaviors towards peers, may be devoting more attention to their warm, supportive mothers at the expense of their peers.

Similar patterns are evident at five. Mothers who were warm at two had children who were more responsive to peers at five. Encouraging perspective taking and using of soft control at two was associated with a child's responsiveness to mother at five. Mothers who exhibit these positive social behaviors were generally more likely to be the targets of more receptive and prosocial behaviors from their children. Positive and prosocial interactions may be one basis for the development of the early social relationship between mother and child as well. The patterns established in this earliest of social relationships between mother and child may then expand to other social relationships with peers and other adults. Thus, the pattern of findings is consistent with previous findings suggesting that maternal warmth, nurturance, expression of affect, and rational direction of the child's behavior are associated with increased social and prosocial behavior (Baumrind, 1971; Bryant & Crockenberg, 1980; Feshbach, 1978; Grusec & Dix, 1986; Rutherford & Mussen, 1968; Yarrow, Scott & Waxler, 1973).

There is less evidence for suggesting a relationship between mother's attitudes or behaviors and the child's social-cognitive processes. The only significant relationship between the child's performance on the perspective taking tasks at two and the mother's behavior was a negative correlation with mother's use of perspective taking in her social interactions with her child. Perhaps the mother's frequent adjustment to the child's perspective decreased the need or opportunity for the child to consider the perspective of the dominant social partner in the early years, the mother. The mother's social behaviors were also not significantly related to the child's empathic responses at five.

Although early prosocial behaviors appear to lack organization or stability, relationships between social-cognitive processes and prosocial behavior across this period suggest that these early behaviors are important for later development. Performance on the perspective-taking tasks was unrelated to social behaviors at two and the measures of empathy were unrelated to responsivity or the composite measures of prosocial behavior, but the child's behaviors at two related to behaviors at five. Prosocial behavior to peers at five was predicted by the quality of attachment at two. Responsiveness to peers at two was significantly related to response to the emotional cues in the empathy stimuli at five, emotional matching and affective empathy. Early skills in perspective taking may be a precursor to responding to situational empathy cues at five. Situational empathy assessed at five was also related to one of the components of prosocial responses at five, compassion. The early social relationships with mother or with peers may not be stable but they do relate to subsequent social behaviors and social skills.

Conclusions

There may be patterns established as early as two years of age which have consequences for later behavior. Mother-child interactions may be a model for later social development with the quality of this relationship, reflected in the warmth and rational guidance of the mother and the attachment relationship, fostering child-mother as well as later child-peer interactions. The mediational role of social-cognitive processes such as perspective taking is less clear. While these processes do not appear to have direct relationships to social behaviors, the early elements of these processes are evident in these young children and the social and social-cognitive experiences of these children contribute to their development.

It is difficult to assess social and social-cognitive processes in young children. Limitations in measurement, particularly for structured measures of socio-cognitive processes in young children, and in sample size need to be considered in these conclusions. The patterns reported here are consistent with previous observational and experimental studies of this age group (Abraham et al., 1983; Baumrind, 1971; Biron et al., 1977; Bryant & Crockenberg, 1980; Feshbach, 1978; Jensen et al., 1981; Rutherford & Mussen, 1968; Yarrow et al., 1973; Zahn-Waxler et al., 1979). These findings expand on previous work in that longitudinal relationships are identified and the role of social experience in the development of social-cognitive processes is demonstrated.

Further exploration of the role of the quality of the early mother-child relationship for subsequent social development is needed. Longitudinal studies with large, diverse samples are needed to replicate these findings and to study the long-term consequences of early patterns of social behavior and of the early mother-child relationship for peer- and parent-child relations into the adolescent years and early adulthood.

References

Abraham, K. G., Kuehl, R. O., & Christopherson, V. A. (1983). Age-specific influence of parental behaviors on the development of empathy in preschool children. *Child Study Journal, 13*, 175-185.

Ahammer, I. M., & Murray, J. P. (1979). Kindness in the kindergarten: The relative influence of role playing and prosocial television in facilitating altruism. *International Journal of Behavioral Development, 2*, 133-157.

Ainsworth, M.D., Blehar, M.C., Waters, E., & Wall, S. (1978). *Patterns of attachment: A psychological study of the strange situation.*

Baumrind, D. (1971). Current patterns of parental authority. *Developmental Psychology Monographs, 4*(1, pt. 2).

Biron, A., Ramos, F., & Higa, W. R. (1977). Cooperation in children: Social and material rewards. *Psychological Reports, 41*, 427-430.

Block, J. (1965). The child rearing practices report. Institute of Human Development, University of California, Berkeley.

Bretherton, I., & Beeghly, M. (1982). Talking about internal states: The acquisition of an explicit theory of mind. *Developmental Psychology, 18*, 906-921.

Bryant, B. K., & Crockenberg, S. B. (1980). Correlates and dimensions of prosocial behavior: A study of female siblings with their mothers. *Child Development, 51*, 529-544.

Buckley, N., Siegel, L. S., & Ness, S. (1979). Egocentrism, empathy, and altruistic behavior in young children. *Developmental Psychology, 15*, 329-330.

Cummings, E. M., Iannotti, R. J., & Zahn-Waxler C. (1985). The influence of conflict between adults on the emotions and aggression of young children. *Developmental Psychology, 21*, 495-507.

Cummings, E. M., Iannotti, R. J., & Zahn-Waxler, C. (1989). Aggression between peers in early childhood: Individual continuity and developmental change. *Child Development, 60*, 887-895.

Deutsch, F. & Madle, R. A. (1975). Empathy: Historic and current conceptualizations, measurement, and a cognitive theoretical perspective. *Human Development, 18*, 267-287.

Devries, R. (1970). The development of role-taking as reflected by behavior of bright, average, and retarded children in a social guessing game. *Child Development, 41*, 759-770.

Dlugokinski, E. L., & Firestone, I. J. (1974). Other centeredness and susceptibility to charitable appeals: Effects of perceived discipline. *Developmental Psychology, 10*, 21-28.

Dunn, J., & Kendrick, C. (1979). Interaction between young siblings in the context of family relationships. In M. Lewis & L. A. Rosenblum (Eds.), *The child and its family.* New York: Plenum Press.

Eckerman, C. O., & Stein, M. R. (1982). The toddler's emerging interactive skills. In K. H. Rubin & H. S. Ross (Eds.), *Peer relationships and social skills in childhood.* New York: Springer-Verlag.

Eisenberg-Berg, N., & Hand, M. (1979). The relationship of preschoolers' reasoning about prosocial moral conflicts to prosocial behaviors. *Child Develoment, 50*, 356-363.

Eisenberg, N., & Lennon, R. (1983). Sex differences in empathy and related capacities. *Psychological Bulletin, 94*, 100-131.

Eisenberg, N., McCreath, H., & Ahn, R. (1988). Vicarious emotional responsiveness and prosocial behavior. *Personality and Social Psychology, 14*, 298-311.

Feshbach, N. D. (1975). Empathy in children: Some theoretical and empirical considerations. *The Counseling Psychologist, 5*, 25-30.

Feshbach, N. D. (1978). Studies of empathic behavior in children. In B. A. Maher (Ed.), *Progress in experimental personality research* (Vol. 8). New York: Academic Press.

Gove, F. L., & Keating, D. P. (1979). Empathic role-taking precursors. *Developmental Psychology, 15*, 594-600.

Grusec, J. E. & Dix, T. (1986). The socialization of prosocial behavior: Theory and reality. In C. Zahn-Waxler, E.M. Cummings, & R. J. Iannotti (Eds.), *Altruism and aggression: Biological and social origins*. New York: Cambridge University Press.

Halperin-Elian, M., & Iannotti, R. J. (1989) Self-referential, empathic, and prosocial behavior in infancy. Paper presented at the meeting of the Society for Research in Child Development, Kansas City.

Hay, D. F. (1979). Cooperative interactions and sharing between very young children and their parents. *Developmental Psychology, 15*, 647-653.

Hoffman, M. L. (1975). Developmental synthesis of affect and cognition and its implications for altruistic motivation. *Developmental Psychology, 11*, 605-622.

Hoffman, M. L., & Levine, L. E. (1976). Early sex differences in empathy. *Developmental Psychology, 12*, 557-558.

Hoffman, M. L., & Saltzstein, H. D. (1967). Parent discipline and the child's moral development. *Journal of Personality and Social Psychology, 5*, 45-57.

Hollingshead, A.B. (1975). Four factor index of social status, Department of Sociology, Yale University.

Iannotti, R. J. (1975). The nature and measurement of empathy in children. *The Counseling Psychologist, 5*(2), 21-24.

Iannotti, R. J. (1977). *A longitudinal investigation of role taking, altruism, and empathy*. Paper presented at the meeting of the Society for Research in Child Development, New Orleans. (ERIC Document Reproduction Service No. ED 136 928)

Iannotti, R. J. (1978). The effect of role-taking experiences on role taking, empathy, altruism, and aggression. *Developmental Psychology, 14*, 119-124.

Iannotti, R. J. (1985). Naturalistic and structured assessments of prosocial behavior in preschool children: The influence of empathy and perspective taking. *Developmental Psychology, 21*, 46-55.

Janssens, J. M. A. M., Gerris, J. R. M., & Janssen, A. W. H. (1989). Childrearing, empathy and prosocial development. Paper presented at the meeting of the Society for Research in Child Development, Kansas City.

Jensen, L., Peery, C., Adams, G., & Gaynard, L. (1981). Maternal behavior and the development of empathy in preschool children. *Psychological Reports, 48*, 879-884.

La Freniere, P.J. (1983). From attachment to peer relations: An analysis of individual differences in preschool peer competence. Paper presented at the meeting of the Society for Research in Child Development, Detroit.

Lamb, M. E., Thompson, R. A., Gardner, W., & Charnov, E. (1985). *Infant-mother attachment: The origins and developmental significance of individual differences in strange situation behavior.* Hillsdale, N.J.: Lawrence Erlbaum Associates Inc.

LeMare, L. J., & Rubin, K. H. (1987). Perspective taking and peer interaction: Structural and developmental analyses. *Child Development, 58*, 306-315.

Lempers, J. D., Flavell, E. R., & Flavell, J. H. (1977). The development in very young children of tacit knowledge concerning visual perspective taking. *Genetic Psychology Monographs, 95*, 3-53.

Liben, L. S. (1978). Perspective-taking skills in young children: Seeing the world through role-colored glasses. *Developmental Psychology, 14*, 87-92.

Londerville, S., & Maine, M. (1981). Security of attachment, compliance, and maternal training methods in the second year of life. *Developmental Psychology, 17*, 289-299.

Mussen, P., & Eisenberg-Berg, N. (1977). *Roots of caring, sharing, and helping.* San Francisco, CA: Freeman.

Pastor, D.L. (1981). The quality of mother-infant attachment and its relationships to toddlers' initial sociability with peers. *Developmental Psychology, 17*, 326-335.

Perry, D. G., Bussey, K., & Freiberg, K. (1981). Impact of adults' appeals for sharing on the development of altruistic dispositions in children. *Journal of Experimental Child Psychology, 32*, 127-138.

Pierrehumbert, B., Iannotti, R. J., Cummings, E. M., & Zahn-Waxler, C. (1989). Social functioning with mother and peers at 2 and 5 years: The influence of attachment. *International Journal of Behavioral Development, 12*, 85-100.

Radke-Yarrow, M., Zahn-Waxler, C., & Chapman, M. (1983). Children's prosocial dispositions and behavior. In P. H. Mussen(Ed.), *Carmichael's manual of child psychology* (Vol. IV, 4th ed.). New York: Wiley.

Rheingold, H. L., Hay, D. R., & West, M. J. (1976). Sharing in the second year of life. *Child Development, 47*, 1148-1158.

Rushton, J. P. (1976). Socialization and the altruistic behavior of children. *Psychological Bulletin, 83*, 893-913.

Rutherford, E., & Mussen, P. (1968). Generosity in nursery school boys. *Child Development, 39*, 755-765.

Shantz, C. U. (1975). Empathy in relation to social cognitive development. *The Counseling Psychologist, 5*, 18-21.

Staub, E. (1971). The use of role playing and induction in children's learning of helping and sharing behavior. *Child Development, 42*, 805-816.

Stewart, R. B., & Marvin, R. S. (1984). Sibling relations: The role of conceptual perspective-taking in the ontogeny of sibling caregiving. *Child Development, 55,* 1322-1332.

Underwood, B., & Moore, B. (1982). The generality of altruism in children. In N. Eisenberg (Ed.), *The development of prosocial behavior.* New York: Academic Press.

Yarrow, M R., Scott, P. M., & Waxler, C.Z. (1973). Learning concern for others. *Developmental Psychology, 8,* 240-260.

Yarrow, M. R., & Waxler, C. Z. (1976). Dimensions and correlates of prosocial behavior in young children. *Child Development, 47,* 118-125.

Zahn-Waxler, C., Radke-Yarrow, M., & Brady-Smith, J. (1977). Perspective-taking and prosocial behavior. *Developmental Psychology, 13,* 87-88.

Zahn-Waxler, C., Radke-Yarrow, M., & King, R. A. (1979). Child rearing and children's prosocial initiations toward victims of distress. *Child Development, 50,* 319-330.

T.G. Power & S.H. Manire

Child Rearing and Internalization: A Developmental Perspective

Central to most theories of socialization and social development is the institution of the family. Sociologists, anthropologists, psychologists, and others have long recognized the important role of families in the early training of cultural norms, beliefs, and values. Despite this intense interest, empirical investigations of the *specific* ways in which cultural transmission occurs in families is still rather limited. The purpose of the present chapter is to summarize some recent descriptive work on this issue, and to present a social-psychological model of the early socialization process. Although this analysis focuses on white, middle-class, American families, many of the concepts and conclusions are general enough to apply to other types of families as well.

Socialization Goals in Middle-Class American Families
An important way that cultural values are transmitted to children is through the realization of parental childrearing goals (Ogbu, 1981; Schaffer, 1984). Although child-rearing goals are influenced by the parent's general socialization values, child-rearing goals are more specific. They refer to the specific characteristics or traits that parents try to encourage or discourage in their children through specific child-rearing interactions.

Previous empirical research on parental child-rearing goals is hard to find. With the exception of some pioneering work by Stoltz (1967) and Kohn (1969) in the 1950's, and the work of Block (1973) in the early 1970's, there has been little systematic study of parental socialization goals and values; instead most research to date has been on child-rearing techniques, i.e., *how* parents achieve their child-rearing goals, not *what* they try to achieve. Therefore, the purpose of our initial research in this area was to identify the range of child-rearing goals that parents attempt to realize in everyday parent-child interactions.

Descritive studies. Data on mothers' and fathers' socialization goals were collected in three studies. In the first (Power & Parke, 1986), 24 families of first-born children (four boys and four girls at each of three ages: 11, 14, and 17 months) were observed in their homes in the hour following dinner. For 45 minutes, observers kept a written record of all parental attempts to influence child behavior, including a description of the specific child behaviors that the parent was trying to influence or elicit. In a follow-up study of 42 families (Power, McGrath, Hughes, & Manire, 1987), mothers and fathers of seven boys and seven girls at two, four, and six years of age were observed. In this study, observations were conducted on two separate evenings from the beginning of dinner until bedtime. To provide additional information on child-rearing practices, parent-child interactions were audio-taped, and separate mother and father interviews were conducted. In the third study (Power & Shanks, 1989), mothers and fathers of 5th, 8th, and 11th graders (seven boys and seven girls at each grade level) were interviewed separately about their child-rearing practices using the interview employed with the parents of preschoolers (Power et al., 1987). Demographically, families in the three studies were similar. Parents were white and middle- to upper-middle class; virtually all parents had at least some college, and about half of the mothers worked full- or part-time outside of the home.

Although many types of child-rearing goals were identified in these studies, parents appeared to have one overriding concern: that their children show general respect for and cooperation with parental authority. This was evidenced by the finding that some of the most severe discipline was used in response to child defiance—independent of the severity of the initial child transgression. Additionally, when an independent sample of 49 mothers of preschoolers rated the severity of the transgressions observed in the Power et al. (1987) study, transgressions involving definace toward authority were rated as among the most severe (Power, Ritter, Bourg, Kelley, & Porfillio, 1987). Only lying and transgressions involving physical harm to the child or others received higher severity ratings.

It is not surprising that instilling respect for authority was such a high priority for these parents. The entire socialization process depends upon its establishment. For parents to achieve *any* socialization goals, their children must cooperate with their demands. Without compliance or cooperation, socialization would be next to impossible.

Our observations and interviews also helped identify some of the more *specific* socialization goals of these white, middle-class Americans (see Table 1). Socialization goals fell into two general categories after Bakan (1966): agency (doing for the self) and communion (doing for others). Child-rearing goals were accomplished in two ways: a) by encouraging or discouraging behaviors that *directly* affected others, such as sharing and aggression; and b) by enforcing household rules that protected the child, others, or their possessions from unintentional physical, psychological, or social harm (such as curfews or limits on child play).

Table 1   Socialization Goals in White, Middle Class American Families

I. *Doing for the Self* (Agency)	II. *Doing for Others* (Communion)
A. Self-Protection	A. Other-Protection
B. Self-Sufficiency	B. Concern for Others
1. Self-Care	1. Kindness/Consideration
2. Independence	2. Cooperation
	3. Altruism/Self-Sacrifice
C. Initiative	C. Manners
1. Striving (i.e., working hard toward goals)	1. Offensive Behavior
2. Assertiveness	2. Deference to Authority
3. Sociability	3. Politeness
D. Competence	D. Integrity
1. Intelligence	1. Honesty
2. Creativity	2. Responsibility
3. Effectiveness	
E. Self-Satisfaction	
1. Emotional Maturity	
2. Psychological Adjustment	

Closer examination of the data showed that with just a few exceptions, the amount of time devoted to three general types of socialization issues was about the same regardless of child age. In each study, about half of the interactions mentioned or observed involved the enforcement of household rules to prevent unintentional harm to the self or others, about one quarter involved encouraging self-sufficiency and independence, and about one-quarter involved encouraging appropriate or responsible interpersonal behavior.[1]

Developmental trends. Examination of the issues common to each study, as well as significant age differences *within* studies, revealed differences that appeared to be a function of child age. Parents of toddlers stressed the enforcement of household rules to prevent harm to the child or others; parents of preschoolers focused on encouraging responsible interpersonal behavior and manners; parents of children in middle childhood encouraged assertiveness and initiative; and parents of adolescents focused on independence, initiative, and household rules regarding possible harm to the child outside of the home.

Thus, with child development, parents appeared to shift back and forth between encouraging behavior that benefited the self and behavior that benefited others. During toddlerhood, parents encouraged self-protection; during the preschool years, they encouraged sacrificing individual needs for the sake of others. In middle childhood, the pendulum swang back again as parents encouraged doing for the self in social situations, and remained there during adolescence when the focus was on independence and self-protection. These differences, of course, were all a matter of degree. At *all* ages, parents encouraged self-serving and other-serving behavior in their children.

Why this particular sequence? The answer probably lies in the egoistic nature of the young child. Parents of young children must temper their child's egoism with the early lessons of socialization, but once these are mastered, they must eventually encourage self-serving behavior to ensure the child's successful adaptation to the competitive American culture. However, now that the foundation for socially responsible behavior has been built, children can be taught to meet their own needs in responsible, socially-appropriate ways.

---

1. Because the focus of these studies was on behavioral rather than cognitive socialization, observational data was not collected on interactions in the competence area in Table 1. If these interactions had been included, these percentages would have been somewhat different.

Socialization Techniques in Middle-Class American Families

In contrast to the literature on socialization issues, considerable attention has been devoted to the study of socialization techniques. By interviewing and/or observing parents and children, researchers have identified a number of commonly-occurring child-rearing styles (e.g, Baldwin, Kalhorn, & Breese, 1945; Baumrind, 1967, 1971; Becker, 1964; Maccoby & Martin, 1983; Schaefer, 1959), as well as commonly used parenting strategies (e.g., Bearison & Cassel, 1975; Hess & Shipman, 1967; Hoffman, 1977).

Although these studies provide important data on individual differences in parenting, they do not describe the *wide range* of techniques that parents use in socializing their children. This is so because researchers have generally focused on parent behavior in only a limited number of child-rearing situations—primarily teaching situations and parental responses to child transgressions. Although much empirical data have been collected to illustrate the importance of these experiences, little is known about the socialization that occurs during more frequent kinds of everyday parent-child interactions.

Schaffer & Crook (Schaffer, 1977, 1984; Schaffer & Crook, 1978) have proposed a method for studying such parenting practices. They argue that instead of providing global descriptions of important variations in child-rearing style, that researchers should broaden their focus to describe the wide range of ways that parents elicit, inhibit, influence, or otherwise control their child's behavior during day-to-day parent-child interactions. By so doing, it is possible to be more specific about the ways that parents achieve their child-rearing aspirations and goals.

Descriptive studies. Schaffer & Crook (1979, 1980) illustrated the utility of their approach in a descriptive study of mothers instructed to actively guide their 15- to 24-month-old's toy play in a laboratory setting. Three subsequent studies in lab and home settings (Power, 1985; Power & Parke, 1982, 1983) traced the origins of these socializing practices in infancy, and demonstrated that parental controls frequently occurred in the absence of specific instructional sets.

More extensive data on parental socialization techniques were collected in two of the studies described above (Power, McGrath et al., 1987; Power & Shanks, 1989). From the home observations and parent interviews, four general types of socialization techniques were identified: situational management, modeling, commands/explanations, and rewards/punishments. Definitions and examples of the techniques identified in each category are presented in Table 2.

Table 2   Child-rearing Techniques in White, Middle Class American
           Families

I. *Situational Management*

  A. *Provide Opportunities*
Structuring child's environment to provide opportunities for desired
behavior or to prevent undesired behavior from occurring in the first
place (e.g., inviting children over for child to play with, enrolling child
in various extracurricular activities, putting dangerous objects out of
sight so that child will not be tempted to touch them).

  B. *Force Compliance*
Forcing compliance through physical intervention (e.g., carrying child
to bed, taking forbidden object from child, stopping fight by separating
children, turning off television or stereo).

II. *Modeling*

Providing a model of socially appropriate behavior through parent's
own actions (e.g., setting example of good table manners, modeling
kindness and cooperation).

III. *Commands/Explantions*

  A. *Tell/Ask*
Telling or asking child to do or not to do something without elaboration (e.g., command, suggest, request, hint, remind).

  B. *Repeat Command*
Repeating telling or asking child to do or not to do something.

  C. *Demonstrate/Instruct*
Teaching child *how* to perform appropriate behavior by direct demonstration, assistance, or instruction (e.g., showing child how to use knife
and fork, helping child make bed, helping child do laundry).

  D. *Reason/Persuade*
Explaining to child *why* he or she should or should not do something
(e.g., explaining consequences of child's actions, providing information about the feelings or thoughts of others, providing information
about child's own past behavior).

Table 2   Continued

IV. *Rewards/Punishments*

A. *Rewards*
1. *Praise*
Praising child to encourage appropriate behavior.
2. *Materially Reward*
Giving child material rewards for engaging in appropriate behavior (e.g., giving child money or a toy, giving child a snack or dessert).
3. *Grant Privileges*
Granting child privileges for engaging in appropriate behavior (e.g., taking child to a movie, allowing child to stay up an hour later than usual).

B. *Punishments*
1. *Scold*
Scolding child to discourage inappropriate behavior.
2. *Ignore*
Ignoring child to discourage inappropriate behavior.
3. *Materially Punish*
Taking away something material from child for engaging in inappropriate behavior (e.g., taking away allowance for a week, taking toy away from child, withholding dessert already promised).
4. *Send to Room*
Sending child to his or her room for engaging in inappropriate behavior.
5. *Physically Punish*
Physically punishing child (e.g., spanking, wrist slapping, hitting child with object).
6. *Deprivation of Privileges/Assign Additional Chore*
Depriving child of privileges or assigning additional chores for engaging in inappropriate behavior (e.g., taking away television privileges, not letting child visit friend, having child clean garage).

Examination of the frequency which parents used the various techniques showed that the conclusions drawn varied as a function of the method of data collection. During the interivews, parents reported the frequent use of reasoning, instruction, and external rewards and punishments. In contrast, during the observations, over 90% of all child-rearing techniques were verbalizations only, with the vast majority being commands, requests, and suggestions (reasoning and instruction were used in only about one-fifth of all control attempts).

Only about two percent of the total observed techniques involved the threat or promise of an external punishment or reward (i.e., materially reward, grant privilege, materially punish, send to room, physically punish, or deprivation of privileges), and in only 9 out of 84 two- to three-hour home observations did the actual administration of an external punishment occur. The overt use of praise\scold was rare as well—together these techniques accounted for about three percent of the total.

The substantial differences between the the interview and observational findings regarding parenting techniques appeared to be a function of the *issues* addressed by these two methods. In the interviews, parents described how they dealt with a wide range of socialization issues including frequent (e.g., finishing dinner, getting ready for bed) and relatively infrequent behaviors (e.g., physical aggression, name-calling, lying). During the observations, parents were observed encouraging or discouraging more common, everyday behaviors such as table manners, self-care skills, and adherence to household rules. When the technique measures were adjusted to make them comparable in terms of the socialization issues being addressed, significant, moderate, positive correlations between the observational and interview measures were found (see Power, McGrath et al., 1987).

An important implication of these findings is that in spite of the fact that parents occasionally used external rewards and punishments to socialize their children, the vast majority of child-rearing techniques during day-to-day socialization interactions were verbal commands, suggestions, requests, and reminders, along with occasional reasoning and instruction. Even these middle- to upper-middle class, college-educated parents (who for the most part would be classified as authoritative), spent most of their time directing their child's behavior with little child input into the socialization process, and with the limited use of reasoning and external motivators. Children were for the most part compliant to their parents' demands. Analyses of the preschool data showed that at each age, about one-half of all parental control attempts were followed by child compliance. In most cases, parents simply told their child what to do or not to do and after zero, one, or two repetitions, the child usually complied. However, often embedded in the repeated parental requests and commands were implicit threats subtly (and sometimes not so subtly!) conveyed in slight variations in wording and voice tone. Thus, at least during everyday interactions with their children, middle-class, American parents do not typically achieve compliance through high-power, external techniques such as power assertion and explicit love withdrawal (e.g., Hoffman, 1977). Instead parents appear to make use of subtle variations in the nature of their verbal requests and directives.

Developmental trends. Examination of the preschool and adolescent data provided some preliminary information on developmental changes in parenting techniques. Parents of two-year-olds forced compliance significantly more often than did parents of four- and six-year-olds (interview and observation data), and parents of two-year-olds were also more likely to use praise and affection (interview and observation data), demonstration and assistance (observation data), and the repetition of commands (observation data). Parents of four- and six-year-olds were more likely to simply tell or ask the child to do or not to do something (interview data), and parents of six-year-olds were more likely to use reasoning and persuasion (observation data). Analyses of the nature of parent justifications (observation data), showed that parents of four- and six-year-olds were more likely to make references to parental authority, to child feelings (mothers only), and to child behavior in the past. Parents of two-year-olds made relatively more references to the likely consequences of child actions.

In adolescence, forcing compliance was most common among parents of eighth graders, and the use of reasoning/persuasion significantly increased with age. Parents of preschoolers were more likely to report sending children to their room and using physical punishment; parents of adolescents were more likely to report providing opportunities and depriving the child of privileges.

These results replicate the findings of previous studies conducted in the 1940's and 1950's in showing that between the ages of three and nine, parents show a decrease in the amount of interaction, stimulation, and discipline (Baldwin, 1946; Clifford, 1959; Lasko, 1954), rely less on situational management (i.e., diverting the child's attention and forcibly removing the child from situations—Clifford, 1959), and show less warmth, indulgence, and protectiveness (Baldwin, 1946; Lasko, 1954). One study using a parent disciplinary diary found that as children got older, parents were less likely to use physical punishment and isolation, and more likely to take away privileges (Clifford, 1959).

Although preliminary, the data support a developmental model of child-rearing originally proposed by Sears, Maccoby, & Levin (1957) and elaborated on in our own work. With increasing child age, parents provided children with increasing opportunities for self-regulation and control, thus making them more and more responsible for their own behavior (see also Bruner, 1978; Kaye, 1982; Kopp, 1982). As outlined by Sears et al. (1957), parental control practices shifted from direct, external controls (e.g., force compliance, demonstrate/assistance) to indirect, external controls (e.g., praise and affection) to the encouragement of internal controls (e.g., reasoning and persuasion). How do these early socialization experiences culminate in the development of internalized, socially responsible behavior? We now turn to a brief presentation of a social-psychological model of the internalization process.

Child-rearing and Internalization: A Developmental Model
Socialization and internalization. Recently, there has been an increased interest among social and developmental psychologists in the concept of internalization (e.g., Grusec, 1983; Hoffman, 1983; Lepper, 1983; Perry & Perry, 1983). Internalization, often contrasted with compliance, refers to the complex psychological process through which children gradually acquire cultural customs and norms, and use them in guiding their behavior, even in the absence of adult supervision and monitoring. The difference between compliance and internalization concerns its motivation: in compliance, children are motivated by expectations for external rewards and punishments; in internalization, the motivation is internal, such as self-induced guilt after deviation or self-induced pleasure and pride after conforming.

A three-component model. In the proposed model, internalization is broken down into three components: a) an understanding of the rules that define appropriate or responsible child behavior in various contexts, b) the ability to exercise sufficient impulse control and self-regulation to follow these rules, and c) the development of an internal versus an external motivation to comply. Although each component makes an individual contribution to the development of internalized, socially responsible behavior, all three are necessary, at least in rudimentary form, for internalization to occur. Because development in each of these areas is gradual during childhood, internalization should be gradual as well. Moreover, it is proposed that parents encourage the development of internalization when their socialization practices contribute to development in any of these areas.

Social understanding. In the present formulation, social understanding refers to the child's understanding of the appropriateness, desirability, or acceptability of a given act or series of actions in a particular context. Social understanding refers to knowledge in a variety of domains. As outlined in Table 1, these include social conventions (manners), moral issues (integrity and concern for others), household rules (self- and other-protection), and expectations for self-sufficiency and self-fulfillment (initiative, competence, self-satisfaction). Moreover, the domain of an issue determines the metric by which it is judged. For example, moral issues require judgments of right and wrong, social conventions require judgments of social appropriateness, and self-sufficiency or self-fulfillment issues require evaluations of success, competence, and care. Thus, not only do children need to learn about right and wrong, they need to differentiate between the various domains of activity that require various judgments.

How do children acquire such knowledge? Unfortunately, very little is known. As is true of cognitive development research in general (cf., Sternberg, 1984), most research into children's social cognition (e.g., Damon, 1977; Kohlberg, 1969; Piaget, 1932; Rest, 1983; Shantz, 1983) has focused on age-related changes in the nature of social knowledge and social cognition, rather than on the acquisition processes themselves. However, some tentative speculations can be offered. Given the young child's curiosity and insatiable desire to learn, it is likely that children acquire social knowledge in the same way that they acquire other types of knowledge: through the active construction of a knowledge base derived through experience (e.g., diSibio, 1982; Nelson, 1986; Piaget, 1977). Environmental input into this system comes in at least two forms: a) exposure to social rules through the verbalizations of others, and b) exposure through the enforcement of social rules in the child's presence. The first source involves information received through direct tuition (reasoning and instruction by socialization agents) or through witnessing verbalizations regarding others (e.g., hearing conversations between socializing agents and children in school, in the homes of their friends, in their own homes regarding siblings, or on television). Because young children do not always understand what they are told, their constructions are likely to be personal and unique—the result of a complex interaction between their cognitive abilities, existing knowledge, biases in social perception, and cumulative experience.

The second source of knowledge comes from children's observation of social rule enactment, primarily observations of the consequences of actions in various situations. Thus, children learn which behaviors are appropriate or inappropriate in a given situation based upon the reactions of others. These consequences need not be imposed by socializing agents. For example, a child can learn that lying is wrong based upon the socializing reactions of parents (e.g., reasoning, scolding, punishment), or upon the normal reactions of others (e.g., peers who become distrustful of a dishonest child). Of course in either situation, alternative, even anitsocial norms may be endorsed (e.g., the adolescent in a youth gang).

What is the range of family socialization experiences relevant to the acquisition of social knowledge? Beyond the descriptive data offered above, very little is known. This is the case even for analyses of reasoning, because with but a few exceptions (e.g., Henry, 1980), researchers have coded reasoning in an undifferentiated and global way. Some tentative speculations, however, can be offered.

Because much of social knowledge involves learning rules that define the appropriateness of self-serving and other-serving behavior in various situations, the tendency of parents to shift back and forth between these two areas throughout development probably facilitates the acquisition of some of the more complex social rules. For example, the egoistic toddler is taught that physical aggression is wrong (concern for others), but once this has been learned, the slightly older child is taught that it is sometimes allowed, but only in self-defense (concern for the self). As the child gets older still, he or she may be taught that aggression is allowed in self-defense, but only as a last resort (concern for others). Thus, by carefully building on the child's developing social knowledge, the understanding of complex social rules can be encouraged.

Despite the relative lack of descriptive data, there is considerable evidence to support the hypothesis that children exposed to greater amounts of social information show greater levels of responsible, socially appropriate behavior. Specifically, parents who use reasoning and persuasion, who communicate clear socialization and maturity demands, and who are consistent in their discipline have children who are the most likely to show socially responsible behavior in their parents' absence (e.g., Baumrind, 1967, 1971; Hoffman & Saltzstein, 1967; Kobayashi-Winata & Power, 1989; Lytton, 1977; Manire & Power, 1983; Slater & Power, 1987). Thus, not only must the child be made aware of social rules and the reasons behind them, the rules must be consistently enforced. When parents are inconsistent, and the enforcement of rules varies across situations, it is difficult for the child to ascertain what the rules actually are.

Ability. The second component of internalization is the ability to regulate one's behavior in response to societal demands. Theorists from very different perspectives argue that this process develops gradually and plays a central role in the development of mature, socialized behavior (e.g., Aronfreed, 1969; Freud, 1955; Kopp, 1982; Vygotsky, 1978). The gradual development of self-regulation has been demonstrated in numerous studies of behavioral inhibition (Masters & Binger, 1978; Sawin & Parke, 1979, 1980), resistance to temptation (Hartig & Kanfer, 1973), and delay of gratification (Miller, Weinstein, & Karniol, 1978).

As proposed above, the parent's role in encouraging self-regulation is to provide the child with much assistance and guidance during the early years, but to gradually withdraw this support as the child grows older. This gives the child more and more responsibility for behavior with increasing age, and thereby encourages independence and internalization. Unfortunately, however, little data are currently available on how parents provide such assistance to children of different ages.

The relationship between the provision of parental assistance and later internalization is also unclear. Although not confirmed by empirical research, one reasonable hypothesis is that some intermediate level of assistance and guidance is the most beneficial. For example, in infancy, Hunt (1961) has argued that optimal development is most likely if there is a "match" between the child's capabilities and the child's environment. Similarly, based upon the writings of Vygotsky (1978), Wertsch (1979) has argued that in teaching situations, successful parents give the child just enough structure to approach a problem, but not so much as to interfere with independent problem solving. He argues that sensitive and effective parents gradually withdraw their support as the child gets older, so as to not interfere with the child's developing competence.

Data from a study by Manire & Power (1983) are consistent with this formulation. In an observational/interview study of five- to six-year-olds, parents who relied on direct-external child-rearing practices at home (such as forcing compliance or preventing behaviors from occurring in the first place) had children who were the least well-behaved at achool. Similar results were obtained by Kobayashi-Winata & Power (1989) in a study of Japanese and American families living in Houston. One interpretation of these findings is that by providing too much direct stucture and guidance in the home, parents may interfere with the development of the self-regulatory abilities required for socially appropriate behavior in the parents' absence. Clearly more work on this issue is needed.

Internal motivation. Finally, for internalization to occur, children must develop an internal rather than an external motivation to comply to societal demands. Knowing what is appropriate and having the ability to act accordingly is clearly not enough: children must be motivated to follow societal rules even in situations where there are pressures to transgress and socializing agents are not present. This should occur when children adopt societal rules as their own and act accordingly, not comply because of the anticipated reactions of others.

Based upon this assumption, it could be predicted that parents who rely primarily on external rewards and punishments to ensure compliance should have children who show the lowest levels of internalization. This is indeed the case. Numerous studies show a negative correlation between the use of power assertive techniques and independently observed measures of socially responsible behavior in the parent's absence (Baumrind, 1967, 1971; Kobayashi-Winata & Power, 1989; Maccoby & Martin, 1983; Manire & Power, 1983; Power & Chapieski, 1986; Rollins & Thomas, 1979).

Although the parenting practices that contribute to an external motivation to comply seem rather obvious, what facilitates the development of an internal motivation? At least four socialization practices appear relevant. First, because many social rules involve considering the welfare of others, socialization practices that encourage empathetic responses in children may be particularly effective in encouraging an internal motivation for socially responsible behavior. In fact, the results of numerous correlational (Dlugokinski & Firestone, 1974; Hoffman, 1960; Zahn-Waxler, Radke-Yarrow, & King, 1979) and experimental (Eisenberg-Berg & Geisheker, 1979; Kuczynski, 1982, 1983; Perry, Bussey, & Freiberg, 1981; Sawin & Parke, 1980) studies support this notion.

A second source of internal motivation is suggested by Lepper (1983). He argues that internal motivations are most likely when socializing techniques are "minimally sufficient" to ensure compliance. That is, the techniques are powerful enough to produce compliance, but are also sufficiently subtle enough to prevent the child from attributing his or her behavior to an external source. This is important, because once an external cause has been identified, internal causes are generally discounted (Dix & Grusec, 1983; Kelley, 1973) and behavior thus comes under external control. If external forces are subtle, behavior is attributed to internal sources, thus leading to internalization (Grusec, 1983; Lepper, 1983).

Lepper (1983) suggests several ways in which subtle social control might be administered by parents. These include: a) suggestive versus directive control attempts, b) modeling of appropriate behavior, c) sharing socialization tasks with the child, and d) statements to increase the child's intrinsic interest in a task. Correlational studies of parents and children provide some support for the effectiveness of the first two strategies (e.g., Averill & Power, 1990; Bee, 1967; Bourg & Power, 1985, 1986; Bryan, 1975; Loeb, 1975; Olvera-Ezzell, Power, & Cousins, 1990; Woolger & Power, 1990), and Lepper & Gilovich (1982) present experimental evidence for the last one. Moreover, Grusec, Kuczynski, Rushton, & Simutis (1978) found that when children were subtly induced to engage in prosocial behavior through modeling, they were more likely to attribute their behavior to internal factors than if direct instructions had been used.

A related means for encouraging an internal motivation to comply is suggested by social psychological studies of attitude change (e.g., Calder, Ross, & Insko, 1973; Collins & Hoyt, 1972). In this research, encouraging the perception of choice or control over one's actions leads to greater attitude change than situations where personal control over actions is limited. When children feel that they have acted out of their own desires, they are probably more likely to attribute their behavior to internal motivation than to external demands. In contrast, when forced to comply against their wishes, they may later actively disobey parental directives to restore their lost behavioral freedom (Brehm & Brehm, 1981). We have recently empirically demonstrated the importance of child input or choice in both correlational (Bourg & Power, 1985) and experimental (Bourg & Cohen, 1988; McGrath & Power, 1990) studies.

Finally, parents may encourage an internal motivation for behavior by providing children with internal attributions for their behavior in situations where the causes of their behavior are not that obvious. This has been demonstrated in several experimental studies as well (e.g., Deinstbier, Hillman, Lehnhoff, Hillman, & Valkennar, 1979; Grusec et al., 1978; Grusec & Redler, 1980).

To what degree do parents use internal versus external techniques to motivate their child's behavior? As described above, parent techniques during our home observations were mostly verbal. Moreover, parents rarely used external rewards and punishments, and relied primarily on verbal requests, suggestions, and commands. Children generally complied without the parent having to resort to high-pressure techniques. According to Lepper's theoretical model of social influence (Lepper, 1983), this situation is ideal for the development of internalization. Because parents reared their children in such a way that children generally complied in the absence of strong external pressures, child behavior should therefore be attributed to more internal than external factors.

Although attribution theory provides a useful perspective on early parental control practices, the contribution of other factors should not be overlooked. Maccoby (1983) argues that children's behavior can be viewed as part of a system of mutual responsiveness and gratification between parent and child. She argues that compliance is most likely when parental requests are part of "a history of joint activity in the pursuit of mutual goals" (p. 369). Consistent with this analysis are the positive correlations generally reported between internalization and parental warmth (Maccoby & Martin, 1983; Rollins & Thomas, 1979).

The quality of the parent-child relationship is important in other ways as well. For example, approval and disapproval can be effective child-rearing practices, because young children generally want to please their parents. This makes it possible to socialize children without relying too heavily on external rewards and punishments. Moreover, if the child grows up in an environment of mutual responsiveness and respect, the child's desire to please and cooperate with the parents may generalize to others, thus providing the basis of an internalized, general concern for others. Given the intense quality of the parent-child bond, further research on its role in motivating internalization is clearly needed.

Conclusions

The proposed model provides many clues as to how parents encourage the development of internalized, socially-responsible behavior in their children. Although the encouragement of such behavior is often difficult—given the numerous, naturally-occurring temptations to transgress—successful parents appear to do the following: a) build the foundation for internalization through the establishment of a warm and supportive parent-child relationship, b) communicate clear expectations for appropriate behavior, c) use only the minimally sufficient external pressure needed to ensure child compliance in given child-rearing situations, and d) instill in their children responsibility for their own behavior by encouraging child input into socialization, and providing the social information needed for children to make responsible, independent decisions. Finally, child-rearing goals and techniques are geared to the developmental level of the child, with parents encouraging increasing child responsibility for behavior as the child matures.

Further research on these issues is clearly needed—on the parenting practices that contribute to internalization, and on developmental changes in parenting practices as well. These issues also need to be considered within a social *interaction* framework since the data presented here only address half of the socialization process—the parent's influence on the child. For example, characteristics of the child undoubtedly influence the socialization issues that parents emphasize, as well as the techniques they employ in the process. This may be particularly true as the child develops, and parents revise and adjust their parenting goals, practices, and values in response to experiences with their children. A more complete understanding of internalization would therefore require detailed analyses of how parental socialization demands are enforced in the context of social interactions, and how children play an active role in their own socialization (Bell & Harper, 1977).

Acknowledgements
The first author would like to express his gratitude to his students for their important contributions to this research program: Louise Andrews, Patricia Averill, Tammy Bourg, Lynn Chapieski, Sheryl Hughes, Michelle Kelley, Hiroko Kobayashi-Winata, Marianne McGrath, Norma Olvera, Alysia Ritter, Sharon Schultz, Josephine Shanks, Belgin Tunali, and Christi Woolger. Many of the ideas in this paper have come out of our extended discussions and our many hours of observing and interviewing parents and children. Much of the research reported here was funded in part by grants from the Foundation for Child Development and from the University of Houston's Student Research Program. Reprint requests should be sent to Thomas G. Power, Psychology Department, University of Houston, Houston, Texas 77204-5341.

References

Aronfreed, J. (1969). The concept of internalization. In D. A. Goslin (Ed.), *Handbook of socialization theory and research* (pp. 263-323). Chicago: Rand McNally.

Averill, P., & Power, T. G. (1990). *The role of parents in sports socialization of six- to eight-year-old boys in soccer.* Unpublished manuscript, University of Houston.

Bakan, D. (1966). *The duality of human existence.* Chicago: Rand McNally.

Baldwin, A. L. (1946). Differences in parent behavior toward three- and nine-year-old children. *Journal of Personality, 15,* 143-165.

Baldwin, A. L., Kalhorn, J., & Breese, F. H. (1945). Patterns of parent behavior. *Psychological Monographs, 58*(3).

Baumrind, D. (1967). Child care practices anteceding three patterns of preschool behavior. *Genetic Psychology Monographs, 75,* 43-88.

Baumrind, D. (1971). Current patterns of parental authority. *Developmental Psychology Monographs, 4*(1, Pt. 2).

Bearison, D. J., & Cassel, T. Z. (1975). Cognitive decentration and social codes: Communication effectiveness in young children from differing family contexts. *Developmental Psychology, 11,* 29-36.

Becker, W. C. (1964). Consequences of different kinds of parental discipline. In M. L. Hoffman & L. W. Hoffman (Eds.), *Review of child development research.* Vol. 1. (pp. 169-208). New York: Russell Sage Foundation.

Bee, H. (1967). Parent-child interaction and distractibility in nine-year-old children. *Merrill-Palmer Quarterly, 13,* 175-190.

Bell, R. Q., & Harper, L. V. (1977). *Child effects on adults.* Hillsdale, NJ: Erlbaum.

Block, J. H. (1973). Conceptions of sex role: Some cross-cultural and longitudinal perspectives. *American Psychologist, 28,* 512-526.

Bourg, T. M., & Cohen, D. (1988, March). *The effects of differentially directive instruction strategies on preschooler's compliance.* Paper presented at the biennial meeting of the Southwestern Society for Research in Human Development, New Orleans.

Bourg, T. M., & Power, T. G. (1985, April). *Maternal strategies for compliance in a resistance to distraction task.* Paper presented at the biennial meeting of the Society for Research in Child Development, Toronto.

Bourg, T. N., & Power, T. G. (1986, March). *The effects of maternal directiveness on child compliance in a resistance to distraction task.* Paper presented at biennial meeting of the Southwestern Society for Research in Human Development, San Antonio.

Brehm, S. S., & Brehm, J. W. (1981). *Psychological reactance: A theory of freedom and control.* New York: Academic Press.

Bruner, J. S. (1978). The role of dialogue in language acquisition. In A. Sinclair, R. J. Jarvella, & W. J. M. Levelt (Eds.), *The child's conception of language.* Berlin: Springer-Verlag.

Bryan, J. H. (1975). Children's cooperation and helping behaviors. In E. Mavis

Hetherington (Ed.), *Review of child development research* (pp. 127-181). Chicago: University of Chicago Press.

Calder,B. J., Ross, M., & Insko, C. A. (1973). Attitude change and attitude attribution: Effects of incentive, choice, and consequences. *Journal of Personality and Social Psychology, 25,* 84-89.

Clifford, E. (1959). Discipline in the home: A controlled observational study of parental practices. *Journal of Genetic Psychology, 95,* 45-82.

Collins, B. E., & Hoyt, M. F. (1972). Personal responsibility-for-consequences: An integration and extension of the "forced compliance" literature. *Journal of Experimental Social Psychology, 8,* 558-593.

Damon, W. (1977). *The social world of the child.* San Francisco: Jossey-Bass.

Deinstbier, R. A., Hillman, D., Lehnhoff, J., Hillman, J., & Valkenaar, M. C. (1979). An emotion-attribution approach to moral behavior: Interfacing cognitive and avoidance theories of moral development. *Psychological Review, 82,* 299-315.

diSibio, M. (1982). Memory for connected discourse: A constructivist view. *Review of Educational Research, 52* 149-174.

Dix, T., & Grusec, J. E. (1983). Parental influence techniques: An attributional analysis. *Child Development, 54,* 645-652.

Dlugokinski, E. L., & Firestone, I. J. (1974). Other-centeredness and susceptibility to charitable appeals: Effects of perceived discipline. *Developmental Psychology, 10,* 21-28.

Eisenberg-Berg, N., & Geisheker, E. (1979). Content of preachings and power of the model/preacher: The effect on children's generosity. *Developmental Psychology, 15,* 168-175.

Freud, S. (1955). Beyond the pleasure principle. In J. Strachey (Ed.), *The standard edition of the complete psychological works. Vol. 18.* (pp. 1-64). London: Hogarth.

Grusec, J. E. (1983). The internalization of altruistic dispositions: A cognitive analysis. In E. T. Higgins, D. N. Ruble, & W. W. Hartup (Eds.), *Social cognition and social development: A sociocultural perspective* (pp. 275-293). Cambridge: Cambridge University Press.

Grusec, J. E., Kucznski, L., Rushton, J. P., & Simutis, Z. M. (1978). Modeling, direct instruction, and attributions: Effects on altruism. *Developmental Psychology, 14,* 51-57.

Grusec, J. E., & Redler, E. (1980). Attribution, reinforcement, and altruism: A developmental analysis. *Developmental Psychology, 16,* 525-534.

Hartig, M., & Kanfer, F. (1973). The role of verbal self instructions in children's resistance to temptation. *Journal of Personality and Social Psychology, 25,* 259-267.

Henry, R. M. (1980). A theoretical and empirical analysis of 'reasoning' in the socialization of young children. *Human Development, 23,* 105-125.

Hess, R.D., & Shipman, V. C. (1967). Cognitive elements in maternal behavior In J. P. Hill (Ed.), *Minnesota symposia on child psychology. Vol. 1* (pp. 57-81). Minneapolis: University of Minneapolis Press.

Hoffman, M. L. (1960). Power assertion by the parent and its impact on the child. *Child Development, 31,* 129-143.

Hoffman, M. L. (1977). Moral internalization: Current theory and research. In L. Berkowitz (Ed.), *Advances in experimental social psychology. Vol. 10* (pp. 85-133). New York: Academic Press.

Hoffman, M. L. (1983). Affective and cognitive processes in moral internalization. In E. T. Higgins, D. N. Ruble, & W. W. Hartup (Eds.), *Social cognition and social development: A sociocultural perspective* (pp. 236-274). Cambridge: Cambridge University Press.

Hoffman, M. L., & Saltzstein, H. (1967). Parent discipline and the child's moral development. *Journal of Personality and Social Psychology, 5,* 45-57.

Hunt, J. McV. (1961). *Intelligence and experience.* New York: Ronald.

Kaye, K. (1982). *The mental and social life of babies: How parents create persons.* Chicago: The University of Chicago Press.

Kelley, H. H. (1973). The processes of causal attribution. *American Psychologist, 28,* 107-128.

Kobayashi-Winata, H., & Power, T. G. (1989). Childrearing and compliance: Japanese and American families in Houston. *Journal of Cross-Cultural Psychology, 20,* 333-356.

Kohn, M. L. (1969). *Class and conformity: A study in values.* Chicago: Dorsey Press.

Kohlberg, L. (1969). Stage and sequence: The cognitive developmental approach to socialization. In D. Goslin (Ed.), *Handbook of socialization research* (pp. 347-480). Chicago: RandMcNally.

Kopp, C. B. (1982). Antecedents of self-regulation: A developmental perspective. *Developmental Psychology, 18,* 199-214.

Kuczynski, L. (1982). Intensity and orientation of reasoning: Motivational determinants of children's compliance to verbal rationales. *Journal of Experimental Child Psychology, 34,* 357-370.

Kuczynski, L. (1983). Reasoning, prohibitions, and motivations for compliance. *Developmental Psychology, 19,* 126-134.

Lasko, J. K. (1954). Parent behavior toward first and second-born children. *Genetic Psychology Monographs, 49.*

Lepper, M. R. (1983). Social-control processes and the internalization of altruistic dispositions: An attributional perspective. In E. T. Higgins, D. N. Ruble, & W. W. Hartup (Eds.), *Social cognition and social development: A sociocultural perspective* (pp. 294-330). Cambridge: Cambridge University Press.

Lepper, M. R., & Gilovich, T. (1982). Activity-oriented request strategies for promoting generalized compliance from children: On accentuating the positive. *Journal of Personality and Social Psychology, 28,* 129-137.

Loeb, R. C. (1975). Concomitants of boys' locus of control examined in parent-child interactions. *Developmental Psychology, 11,* 353-358.

Lytton, H. (1977). Correlates of compliance and the rudiments of conscience in two-year-old boys. *Canadian Journal of Behavioral Sciences, 9,* 242-251.

Maccoby, E. E. (1983). Let's not overattribute to the attribution process: Comments on social cognition and behavior. In E. T. Higgins, D. N. Ruble, & W. W. Hartup (Eds.), *Social cognition and social development: A sociocultural perspective* (pp. 356-370). Cambridge: Cambridge University Press.

Maccoby, E. E., & Martin, J. A. (1983). Socialization in the family: Parent-child interaction. In E. M. Hetherington (Ed.), *Handbook of child psychology. Vol. 4. Socialization, personality, and social development* (pp. 1-101). New York: Wiley. (P. H. Mussen, General Editor)

Manire, S. H., & Power, T. G. (1983, March). *Compliance and the young child: The role of the parents.* Paper presented at the biennial meeting of the Society for Research in Child Development, Detroit.

Masters, J., & Binger, C. (1978). Interrupting the flow of behavior: The stability and development of children's initiation and maintenance of compliant response inhibition. *Merrill-Palmer Quarterly, 24,* 229-242.

McGrath, M. P., & Power, T. G. (1990). The effects of reasoning and choice on children's prosocial behavior. *International Journal of Behavioral Development. 13,* 345-353

Miller, D., Weinstein, S., & Karniol, R. (1978). Effects of age and self-verbalization on children's ability to delay gratification. *Developmental Psychology, 14,* 569-570.

Nelson, K. (1986). *Event knowledge: Structure and function in development.* Hillsdale, N. J.: Lawrence Erlbaum Associates.

Ogbu, J. U. (1981). Origins of human competence: A cultural-ecological perspective. *Child Development, 52,* 413-429.

Olvera-Ezzell, N., Power, T. G., & Cousins, J. H. (1990). Maternal socialization of children's eating habits: Strategies used by obese Mexican-American mothers. *Child Development, 61,* 395-400.

Perry, D. G., Bussey, K., & Freiberg, K. (1981). Impact of adults' appeals for sharing on the development of altruistic dispositions in children. *Journal of Experimental Child Psychology, 32,* 127-138.

Perry, D. G., & Perry, L. C. (1983). Social learning, causal attribution, and moral internalization. In J. Bisanz, G. L. Bisanz, & R. Kail (Eds.), *Learning in children: Progress in cognitive development research* (pp. 105-136). New York: Springer-Verlag.

Piaget, J. (1932). *The moral judgment of the child.* New York: Free Press.

Piaget, J. (1977). *The development of thought: Equilibration of cognitive structures.* New York: Viking.

Power, T. G. (1985). Mother- and father-infant play: A developmental analysis. *Child Development, 56,* 1514-1524.

Power, T. G., & Chapieski, M. L. (1986). Childrearing and impulse control in toddlers: A naturalistic investigation. *Developmental Psychology, 22,* 271-275.

Power, T. G., McGrath, M. P., Hughes, S. H., & Manire, S. H. (1987, April). *Mothers, fathers, and childrearing: Socialization during the preschool years.* Paper presented at the Society for Research in Child Development, Baltimore.

Power, T. G., & Parke, R. D. (1982). Play as a context for early learning: Lab and home analyses. In L. M. Laosa, & I. E. Sigel (Eds.), *Families as learning environments for children* (pp. 147-178). New York: Plenum.

Power, T. G., & Parke, R. D. (1983). Patterns of mother and father play with their eight-month-old infant: A multiple analyses approach. *Infant Behavior and Development, 6,* 453-459.

Power, T. G., Parke, R. D. (1986). Patterns of early socialization: An analysis of mother- and father-infant interaction in the home. *International Journal of Behavioral Development, 9,* 331-341.

Power, T. G., & Ritter, A., Bourg, T. M., Kelley, M., & Porfillio, J. (1987, April). *Maternal evaluations of preschooler's transgressions.* Paper presented at the Society for Research in Child Development, Baltimore.

Power, T. G., & Shanks, J. A. (1989). Childrearing in adolescence: A developmental analysis. *Journal of Youth and Adolescence, 18,* 203-220.

Rest, J.R. (1983). Morality. In J. H. Flavell & E. M. Markman (Eds.), *Handbook of child psychology. Vol. 3. Cognitive development* (pp. 556-629). New York: Wiley. (P. H. Mussen, General Editor).

Rollins, B. C., & Thomas, D. L. (1979). Parental support, power, and control techniques in the socialization of children. In W. R. Burr, R. Hill, F. I. Nye, & I. L. Reiss (eds.), *Contemporary theories about the family. Vol. 1. Research-based theories* (pp. 317-364). New York: Free Press.

Sawin, D., & Parke, R. D. (1979). Development of self-verbalized control of resistance to deviation. *Developmental Psychology, 15,* 120-127.

Sawin, D., & Parke, R. D. (1980). Empathy and fear as mediators of resistance to deviation in children. *Merrill-Palmer Quarterly, 26,* 123-133.

Schaefer, E. S. (1959). A circumplex model for maternal behavior. *Journal of Abnormal and Social Psychology, 59,* 226-235.

Schaffer, H. R. (1977). *Mothering.* Cambridge: Cambridge University Press.

Schaffer, H. R. (1984). *The child's entry into a social world.* London: Academic Press.

Schaffer, H. R., & Crook, C. K. (1978). The role of the mother in early social development. In H. McGurk (Ed.), *Issues in childhood social development* (pp. 55-78). London: Methuen.

Schaffer, H. R., & Crook, C. K. (1979). Maternal control techniques in a directed play situation. *Child Development, 50,* 989-996.

Schaffer, H. R., & Crook, C. K. (1980). Child compliance and maternal control techniques. *Developmental Psychology, 16,* 54-61.

Sears, R. R., Maccoby, E. E., & Levin, H. (1957). *Patterns of childrearing.* Evanston, IL: Row & Petersen.

Shantz, C. U. (1983). Social cognition. In J. H. Flavell & E. Markman (Eds.), *Handbook of child psychology: Cognitive development. Vol. 3* (pp. 495-555). New York: Wiley. (P. H. Mussen, General Editor).

Slater, M. A., & Power, T. G. (1987). Mutidimensional assessment of parenting in single-parent families. In J. P. Vincent (Ed.), Advances in family interaction, assessment, and theory. *Vol. 4.* Greenwich, Conn.: JAI Press.

Sternberg, R. J. (1984). *Mechanisms of cognitive development.* New York: W. H. Freeman.

Stoltz, L. M. (1967). *Influences on parent behavior.* Stanford, CA: Stanford University Press.

Vygotsky, L. S. (1978). *Mind in society: The development of higher psychological processes.* Cambridge, MA: Harvard University Press.

Wertsch, J. V. (1979). From social interaction to higher psychological processes: A clarification of Vygotsky's theory. *Human Development, 22,* 1-22.

Woolger, C., & Power, T. G. (1990, March). Socialization of competitive age-group swimmers: a study of mother and father influences. Paper presented at the Southwestern Society for Research in Human Development, Dallas.

Zahn-Waxler, C., Radke-Yarrow, M., & King, R. A. (1979). Childrearing and children's prosocial initiations toward victims of distress. *Child Development, 50,* 319-330.

L. Kuczynski

The Concept of Compliance
in Child-rearing Interactions

An important advance in our understanding of socialization within the family has been the recent growth of a large body of research on children's compliance or obedience to the requests and prohibitions of their parents. Developmental research on compliance began in the early 1970's (e.g. Stayton, Hogan & Ainsworth, 1971; Lytton, 1980; Minton Kagan & Levine, 1971), a time when researchers began to turn away from global child-rearing outcomes (see Martin, 1975 for review) to observational investigations of discrete parent-child interactions. It is likely that early investigations of compliance were as much fostered by the requirements of observational methodology as they were by theoretical considerations. Unlike abstract constructs such as internalization, immediate compliance provided a frequent, observable and easy to define gauge of the outcomes of parent-child interactions. A second body of research concurrently developed in behavior modification treatment interventions and research with aggressive and oppositional children who displayed dysfunctional levels of noncompliance. (e.g. Forehand 1977; Patterson, 1982; Patterson, DeBarsyshe, & Ramsey, E. (1989). The importance of immediate compliance as a child-rearing construct was particularly enhanced in Patterson's work where it is described as a key criterion of parental effectiveness and of child adjustment.

A purpose of this paper is to explore the conceptualizations of immediate compliance and underlying models of parental skill that are emerging from the developmental and behavior modification literatures. The behavior modification perspective will be described first because it provides a coherent unidimensional conceptualization of compliance that serves as a useful framework with which to view alternative models. It is premature to describe a definitive developmental model because there have been few attempts (e.g. Maccoby & Martin, 1983) to integrate the diverse notions of compliance that have emerged from various areas of developmental research. However, the outlines of important elements of a developmental model are apparent and clearly pose a challenge to the models of compliance and parental skill proposed by behavior modification perspectives. My goal in this chapter is to illustrate how new developmental conceptualizations of obedience and control are taking shape.

Undifferentiated Behavioral Model of Compliance/Noncompliance.
The behavioral formulation of compliance and child management practices that promote it could be described as an undifferentiated "no nonsense" model of compliance/noncompliance. Essentially, compliance is conceptualized as being desirable, and adaptive; noncompliance is viewed as undesirable and maladaptive. Behavioral researchers emphasize the dysfunctional nature of noncompliance and point out that noncompliant behavior is the most frequent reason for clinical referral of young children (Forehand, 1977). Patterson (Patterson, 1982; Patterson, DeBarsyshe, & Ramsey, 1989) in particular, has argued that noncompliance is a coercive, antisocial behavior and implicated noncompliance as a key factor in the development of aggression and delinquency. Steps in the developmental progression proposed by Patterson and his colleagues include: unskilful parental management of noncompliance in the home, conduct disorders in early childhood, academic failure and poor peer relationships in middle childhood, depression, and involvement in deviant peer groups in adolescence and, ultimately, delinquency and a host of other problems in adulthood. In Patterson's conceptualization noncompliance also plays an important role in the dynamics of family interactions that contribute to the long-term maintenance of noncompliance. Frequent noncompliance is assumed to contribute to parental stress which ultimately causes further impairments in parent's ability to manage their children's behavior (Patterson, 1982).

The behavioral conceptualization of compliance/noncompliance is undifferentiated in the sense that noncompliance has no independent meaning from compliance. Operationally, compliance and noncompliance are defined with reference to a single time criterion. Forehand and MacMahon (1981) use 5 seconds after a parental request as a criterion for compliance with young 3-8 year old children whereas Patterson (1982; Patterson and Forgatch, 1987) uses a 12 second criterion for defining compliance in young adolescents. Any other response would be defined as noncompliance.

Furthermore, no distinctions are made among varieties of compliance or different qualities of noncompliance. In behavioral interventions parents are encouraged to adopt a highly generalized conception of noncompliance. In the conceptualization of Patterson and his colleagues, noncompliance is listed as one of a list of 14 coercive behaviors that also include hitting, teasing, destruction, crying. In Forehand and MacMahon's (1981) intervention model parents are encouraged to label a broad range of behaviors as noncompliance—not only failure to carry out an instruction given for the first time but also transgressions against rules and commands that have been given in the past. "The rule has been stated at one point in time and does not have to be repeated daily. Using such a conceptualization of noncompliance, whining, playing with matches, fighting, destroying property, "smart talking" and almost any other deviant behaviour of a young child can be viewed as noncompliance" (Forehand and MacMahon, 1981; p.2).

It is useful to explore some of the implications of this undifferentiated conception. Missing are distinctions among different types of children's transgression or the parental requests. Demands with a "do it now and in my presence" quality and no relevance beyond the immediate situation are not distinguished from issues that have long-term moral implications. No distinctions are made on the basis of the quality of the child's compliance or motivation—whether compliance was willing or coerced. There are no distinctions based on the quality of the child's noncompliant behavior—whether noncompliance was appropriately or inappropriately expressed. Finally there are no distinctions based on developmental considerations. With few exceptions, strategies and expectations appropriate for a 4 year old are considered to be appropriate for a 14 year old.

Given the central role of immediate compliance in behavioral formulations of child-rearing goals, it is not surprising that the behavior modification model of parental skill consists of an undifferentiated power assertive approach. Essentially, parents are taught to use effectively their power and control over their children's resources in order to secure children's compliance with their commands. The particular child management skills that are emphasized vary slightly from program to program and are described in available behavioral parent training manuals (e.g. Forehand & McMahon, 1981; Patterson,1975; Patterson & Forgatch,1987). In general, the programs have the following elements in common: Parents are taught to track noncompliance in their interactions with children and to monitor their children's behavior outside the home; they learn to deliver clear, direct forceful commands; they learn to administer positive reinforcements such as parental attention, praise or material rewards contingent on compliance; they learn to administer punitive consequences such as ignoring, time out, work chores and deprivations of material resources contingent on noncompliance.

The emphasis on external incentives and external controls is particularly striking when it is noted that strategies such as explanations, suggestion, and compromise that decrease the salience of the parent's power or offer the child even an illusion of choice are not only missing from the repertoires of skills offered to parents, but are actively discouraged (Patterson, 1982; Forehand & MacMahon 1981). Reid (1982) for instance, suggests that "Rather than teaching parents to talk and lecture and explain to the young child when they discover transgressions, it is probably the case that they should rely on discipline techniques which quickly terminate the interaction with the child in a manner which gives the parent a feeling of success". The assumption is that explanations are, at best, ineffectual in terms of eliciting immediate compliance and therefore, have little place in parental repertoires of child-rearing skills.

Emerging Developmental Perspectives
Immediate compliance also plays a role in developmental perspectives on child rearing. Many writers (e.g.Baumrind,1971; Lytton, 1980; Maccoby & Martin 1984; Perry & Perry; 1983) argue that children's compliance to external control must not be underestimated. Some level of compliance is important and might underlie further developments in children's social development. Furthermore, the development of the capacity to be externally controlled and to comply immediately with the requests of parents has itself, been found to involve a long, drawn-out process (Kopp, 1982). A contribution of the behavior modification perspective is its demonstration that far from being a "given", the capacity to promote compliance to their external authority is one which many parents have difficulty managing. Nevertheless, developmental researchers have not been as enamoured with immediate compliance as a child-rearing goal as have behavioral researchers. The developmentalist's wariness of obedience and com-

pliance has many sources. Milgram's (1974) studies on the danger's of thoughtless compliance to commands of persons of authority raised the idea that children ought to be inoculated against automatic obedience. The notion that there is a fundamental opposition between compliance and children's developing autonomy is enshrined in the concept of the "terrible two's" and runs throughout the developmental literature on child rearing, moral development, and motivation. Finally, the idea that external control or compliance to pressures of external authorities is an earlier developmental achievement and thus represents a more primitive level of functioning than internal control can be found in the early literatures of internalization (Hoffman, 1970), and moral judgement (Kohlberg, 1969).

Interview studies with parents also suggest that parents have a more ambivalent attitude towards obedience than the behavioral concept of compliance suggests. In several studies, only a minority of mothers reported that they expected children to comply immediately with their requests (Sears, Maccoby & Levin, 1957; Newson & Newson, 1968; Zelkovitz, 1982). These studies suggest that although parents consider immediate compliance very nice to have indeed, immediate compliance represents only one of the issues parents face when they attempt to control their children's behavior. Other issues that have been explored in the developmental research include the problem of fostering children's long-term compliance to certain of their commands, and supporting their children's developing autonomy.

One approach that leads to a more differentiated model of parental control and children's compliance is to consider the motivational bases of children's responses to parental directives. At least three categories of compliance have been distinguished on the basis of children's motivation for following parental directives. These are internally motivated compliance, externally motivated compliance and receptive compliance. Recently, researchers also have begun to examine children's motivations for resisting parental controls and to distinguish among various ways in which noncompliance can be expressed. These distinctions are important because different qualities of compliance and of noncompliance are meaningful in terms of the child's behavior. There is also accumulating evidence that many similar distinctions are made by the parents themselves when interacting with their children. In fact, the ability to adapt strategies to different issues posed by children's behavior may constitute an important element of parental skill (Kuczynski, 1984).

External and Internal Motivations for Compliance
A longstanding motivational distinction in the developmental literature is that between externally motivated compliance and internally
motivated compliance. The original theoretical rationale for this
distinction was adapted from motivational theories of moral internalization (Hoffman,1970; Lepper, 1973; 1982). These theories proposed
that parents who predominately used power-assertive strategies in the
course of disciplining their children hindered the internalization of
moral standards whereas parents who used inductive strategies such
as reasoning or low power strategies that minimize the salience of
parental force facilitate the internalization of moral standards.

An important assumption of internalization theories is that
long-term exposure to a consistent parental disciplinary style will lead
to enduring outcomes in children's moral development. Hoffman's
theory, in particular, conceptualized both parental discipline and
children's internalization in trait-like terms. However, because internalization theories have also included assumptions concerning
children's immediate responses to parental discipline, many of the
concepts found in internalization theory can also be employed to
understand the impact of specific parental interventions on specific
acts of compliance (e.g. Kuczynski, 1982; 1983).

Thus, externally motivated compliance is compliance that is primarily motivated by incentives based on parental use of force or their
control over material resources. From a motivational perspective the
child management strategies taught by behavior modification
approaches to parent training: unexplained commands, rewards,
direct parental force, deprivation of privileges, external monitoring
and surveillance provide the essential ingredients for externally motivated compliance. However, other parental practices such as physical
punishment, verbal abuse, unenforced threats which are considered
harmful or ineffectual from the behavioral perspective are also
included in the naturalistic conception of power assertion.

Internally motivated compliance is primarily maintained by motivational resources residing within the child. Numerous ways of
promoting internally motivated compliance based on minimal use of
power (Lepper, 1973; 1982) character attributions (Grusec & Redler,
1980) enhancing children's autonomy (Eghrari and Deci, 1986) induction and explanation (Hoffman, 1970; Kuczynski, 1982; 1983) have
been presented elsewhere. To simplify the present discussion we will
focus on parent's provision of explanations as a strategy that can
promote internally motivated compliance. Both indirect and direct

processes have been proposed to explain the efffects of reasoning on children's internal motivations. Parental use of explanation may promote internal motivations for compliance indirectly, by making it easier for children to attribute their compliance to internal causes such as personality dispositions (Lepper, 1982). However, some forms of reasoning could also directly arouse internal motivations if they directly appeal to internal motives such as children's self-esteem, guilt or empathy (Hoffman, 1970).

Of course, in actual practice, the amount and type of motivation associated with a particular act of compliance or aroused by a particular disciplinary intervention is difficult to determine. The external power of the parent depends on the consistency with which parents have actually administered threatened or promised consequences in the past. Parents can also continue to exert external control over the child's behavior in their absence if they have demonstrated that they can detect noncompliance either by checking up on the child's performance or other forms of monitoring. Moreover, the amount and quality of internal control produced by an explanation should also vary as a function content of explanation, age of child and other variables (Kuczynski, 1982; 1983). Indeed, some qualities of internal motives might also need to be distinguished. Deci & Ryan (1987) suggest that internal motives themselves have intrapsychic counterparts to internal and external motivation. They distinguish between "internal control"—guilt, self-consciousness, superego involvement (identified by constraining thoughts such as "I should", "I have to")—and "autonomous self-regulation" which is characterized by greater flexibility and absence of internal pressure to conform (identified by thoughts such as "I'd find it valuable to..." or "I'd be interested in..."). Finally, any act of compliance is probably determined by mixtures of internal and external motives. This is likely because parents often use a combination of power assertive and inductive strategies during episodes of discipline in the natural environment (Grusec & Kuczynski, 1980; Kuczynski, 1984; Zahn-Waxler, Radke-Yarrow & King, 1979).

What is important for the present purpose is that the kind of motivation that is aroused by a control intervention has important implications for the characteristics of the compliance to which it is attached. For externally motivated behavior, the amount of control exerted by the socializing agent is unstable and fluctuates over time, varying with children's perception that their noncompliance will be detected. An important consequence is that although externally motivated compliance might be effectively elicited and maintained in the presence of the parent it is not very durable, and tends to decrease over time, especially in the parent's absence. In contrast, the presumed source of control for internally motivated compliance is within the children themselves. This kind of compliance should be more durable in the absence of external surveillance because the parent is no longer the source of control for that behavior.

Empirical evidence for the distinction between relatively durable internally motivated compliance and immediate but less durable externally motivated compliance has been collected almost entirely within the context of laboratory "resistance to deviation" paradigms. In such studies, children's compliance with an experimenter's prohibition is usually measured in the experimenter's absence under conditions where, from children's point of view, there is little risk of being found out. In two important studies (Parke, 1969; Cheyne & Walters, 1969) children's compliance was assessed at three successive points in time during a 15 minute resistance to deviation test. It was found that in the absence of an explanation children compliance to a prohibition declined over time. Children who received a substantial explanation for being required to comply with a prohibition complied at a high and stable rate over time. Leizer and Rogers (1974) tested children's compliance in the socializing agent's absence both immediately and on a two week delayed test and also found that reasoning promoted greater long term-resistance to deviation than a verbal reprimand.

A study by Kuczynski (1983) went a step further by providing an explicit test of the motivational bases of children's compliance. In that study compliance was measured as the amount of external control present in the situation was experimentally manipulated. Three control strategies were compared:1) an other-oriented rationale, a form of reasoning designed to arouse children's empathy for the experimenter by pointing out how noncompliance would affect the experimenter, 2) a self-oriented rationale, a form of reasoning that was designed to sensitize children to the external consequences of noncompliance for themselves and 3) a simple prohibition which offered no explanation for requiring children to comply. Children's compliance to the prohibition was subsequently tested under three successive levels of external control: The first test, in the experimenters' presence, was analogous to naturalistic measures of immediate compliance and was represented compliance under conditions of high external control. The second test in the experimenter's absence was considered to represent an intermediate level of external control, because a degree of control could reside in children's beliefs that, despite appearances to the contrary, their deviation could still be detected. The final test in the experimenter's absence following a disinhibition manipulation was designed to completely eliminate fear of detection as a source of motivation for compliance. This was accomplished when the experimenter returned to inform children that although some work would still be appreciated, he would not be angry if children played with toys during his absence.

The findings are useful in illustrating the important principle that judgements regarding the effectiveness of a control strategy depend on how compliance is defined. In the experimenter's presence, no differences were found between the three types of training. A simple power assertive prohibition was as effective as the other-oriented explanation and more effective than the self-oriented explanation in eliciting children's compliance. However, in the two tests in the experimenter's absence, compliance to the unexplained prohibition and the self-oriented explanation decreased precipitously whereas compliance to the other-oriented prohibition remained stable over time.

This finding helps to put into perspective several observational findings that power assertive strategies are more effective than reasoning in eliciting immediate compliance (e.g. Hetherington, Cox & Cox, 1978; Lytton 1980; Minton, Kagan & Levine, 1971). The simple use of power is sufficient if immediate compliance is the criterion of effectiveness. However, inductive strategies are necessary for compliance that will persist in the parent's absence when the external supports for children's compliance are removed.

An implication of this differentiated view of compliance and one which marks a change in perspective from the early internalization literature is that internally motivated compliance is not considered to be superior to externally motivated compliance. Rather, both have their purposes in the day to day rearing of children. An important consideration is whether parents use the strategies that are appropriate for their goals in specific situations (Kuczynski,1984).

Most of the controls directed by parents to their children during a typical day probably involve issues of short-term compliance. The parent's goals for children are often immediate and situation-specific. Usually they are less interested in exerting a long-term influence over children's behavior than they are in getting their children to do or not do something, immediately and in their presence. An unexplained command or simple assertion of power is sufficient for this purpose.

In less frequent situations, parents do have long-term compliance or even internalization as a goal. Sometimes they do want to exert an enduring control over children's behavior. One class of such situations are those in which moral issues are salient—honesty, harm to others. Another class of situations that are likely to arouse parental goals for long-term compliance are those that have implications for children's physical safety and psychological welfare. When a situation does arouse long-term socialization goals, parents are more likely to use strategies that are intended to promote internal motivations for compliance.

There is evidence that parents in well-functioning families have an implicit understanding of the distinction between long-term compliance and short-term compliance and the strategies necessary to achieve them. In a study by Grusec & Kuczynski (1980) mothers were asked how they would react to 12 hypothetical transgressions by their children. Most of the transgressions elicited power assertive techniques. Examples included fighting with peers, noisiness, playing ball in the living room, ignoring a call to dinner. Reasoning was a predominant strategy after only three transgressions: stealing from mother's purse, teasing an elderly man, and running blindly into the street. One interpretation of this pattern of findings is that stealing, molesting the elderly and running into the street all have long-term implications for the child's well-being. Parents may have used reasoning in these situations in the attempt to exert a long-term influence over these behaviors.

Kuczynski (1984) provided experimental evidence that there are two domains of parental influence strategies related to short-term and long-term compliance goals. Mothers were observed interacting in a laboratory setting in which they were asked to influence their 4-year-old children to work on a monotonous task in the face of distraction from an attractive display of toys. Prior to the interactions, mothers' perceptions of their goal in the interaction were experimentally manipulated. Mothers in the short-term goal condition were lead to believe that the experimenter would be assessing only how much their children complied in the their presence. Mothers in the long-term goal condition were given the additional information that, after a while, they would leave the room and their children's compliance would also be assessed in their absence. This awareness that there were longer term requirements for their children's behavior was assumed to elicit in mothers a goal to exert an influence over their children's behavior that would persist in their absence.

As predicted, mother's perceptions of their goal did influence the kinds of strategies they chose to influence their children's behavior during a subsequent interaction. Mothers in the long-term goal condition spontaneously used a pattern of strategies that included a more nurturant interaction during a preliminary free play session, more reasoning, more positive character attributions and more attempts to engage children in conversation. Mothers in the short-term goal condition tended to rely on power assertion alone as a means of maintaining their children's compliance.

A study by Trickett and Kuczynski (1986) suggested that the ability of parents to discriminate among situations requiring short-term and long-term compliance might be an important aspect of parental skill. In that study the discipline strategies of child abusing parents and a matched sample of non-child-abusing parents were compared. In accord with previous findings, non-abusive parents were found to be highly discriminating in their use of discipline. Non-abusive parents tended to rely on unexplained power assertive strategies for transgressions in which immediate compliance issues were salient such as noisy disruptive behaviors and noncompliance. However, for transgressions that involved issues of long-term compliance—moral transgressions and long standing household rules—nonabusive parents used reasoning and explanation at high rates. In contrast, child-abusing parents were less discriminating in their use of discipline strategies. They used unexplained punishment regardless of the nature of the child's transgression. An implication of this study is that the failure of abusive parents to adapt their strategies to differences in transgression may be maladaptive in terms of their children's socialization because, in effect, they were using strategies with short-term effects for long-term purposes.

Receptive Compliance

A third category of compliance that needs to be mentioned is receptive compliance. This is a term recently proposed by Maccoby and Martin (1983) to describe a form of compliance that stems from a generalized willingness by children to cooperate with their parents. Although receptive compliance can be considered to be a form of what we have called internally motivated compliance, it is reasonable to classify separately because its origins are apparently quite different. The concept of receptive compliance originates in findings from the attachment literature (e.g. Londerville & Main, 1981; Matas, Arend & Sroufe 1978) that children who have received secure attachment ratings show higher rates of immediate compliance that children who receive insecure attachment ratings. Although some psychologists have ascribed this pattern directly to the attachment relationship, other interpretations are possible. 1) It may be that the maternal qualities, sensitivity and receptivity to infant cues, that promote secure attachment may also be responsible for sensitive tracking of children's compliance and skilful use of control strategies. 2) It is also possible that a history of responsive interactions with their mothers can directly generate a willingness in children cooperate with parental instructions.

There is evidence to support this latter interpretation. Several studies (e.g. Stayton, Hogan & Ainsworth, 1971; Lytton, 1980) reported a direct relationship between maternal responsiveness and children's compliance. More recent studies (Parpal & Maccoby, 1985; Lay, Waters & Park, 1989) indicated that relatively short interventions designed to train parents to responsively follow their children's cues during play sessions can enhance children's compliance.

A possibility that remains to be explored is that mothers under some conditions may spontaneously increase their responsivity to children as a kind of control strategy in order to increase their children's receptivity to their subsequent commands. Indirect support for this hypothesis was found in the study reported previously (Kuczynski, 1984). Prior to asking their children to perform an arduous task for them, mothers whose goal was to exert a long-term control over children's behavior spontaneously interacted in a more nurturant, responsive manner with their children during a free play session than mothers in a short-term compliance condition. This enhanced involvement in children's play may have been an attempt to elicit children's receptive compliance.

Noncompliance: Autonomy and Social Skill
As indicated earlier, behavior modification research with aggressive and oppositional children has lead to conceptualizations of noncompliance as an aversive, maladaptive behavior. This notion poses problems for those interested in socialization in well-functioning families because it is clear that nonproblem children also engage in a considerable amount of noncompliance. Studies of nonclinic populations report that children disobey between 20% and 40% of the commands of their parents (Forehand, 1977) and Patterson and

Forgatch (1987) suggest that a noncompliance rate as high as 50% falls within reasonable bounds for 10 to 11 year olds. Clearly, this is too much behavior to understood as a sort of childhood dysfunction!

A recent developmental perspective on children's noncompliance (e.g. Crockenberg & Litman, 1987; Kuczynski, Kochanska, Radke-Yarrow & Girnius-Brown, 1987; Kuczynski & Kochanska, 1990) adopted the developmental perspective that some level of noncompliance to parental authority is a positive sign of children's developing autonomy and assertiveness. The process of children's autonomy development has an early impact on parent-child interactions. There is evidence that by the second year of life when toddlers become more and more *able* to comply (Kopp, 1982; Vaughan Kopp & Krakow, 1984), they also become less and less *willing* to comply. During this time children are thought to develop a sense of independent self and a motive to resist threats to their autonomy. This apparent motivational change is manifested by a period of "negativism" or increased overt and active resistance to parental control (Wenar, 1982). The motive to defend one's autonomy and independence against excessive external control, no doubt, continues beyond the toddler period and underlies phenomena such as "reactance" (Brehm, 1981) and "counter-control" (Mahoney, 1974) throughout childhood, adolescence and beyond. Thus one function of noncompliance in the parent-child relationship is that it may serve as a context for children's development of autonomy.

Using this developmental framework we (Kuczynski *et al.*1987; Kuczynski & Kochanska, 1990) have proposed several differentiations within the noncompliance category. One distinction is between passive noncompliance—ignoring or not responding to a directive, and active noncompliance which is accompanied by signs of deliberate resistance or refusal. We consider passive noncompliance to be a relatively unassertive form of resistance that could serve as an index of children's development as autonomous agents. Consistent with this idea, several studies have found that passive noncompliance becomes replaced by more active forms of resistance during the second and third years of life (Vaughan, Kopp & Krakow, 1984; Kuczynski *et al.*, 1987) and indeed from the toddler period to age 5 (Kuczynski & Kochanska, 1990).

We also made distinctions among children's active noncompliant behaviors (Kuczynski *et al.*, 1987). As we observed children's disobedience from this optimistic perspective it occurred to us that noncompliance might also be a context for children to practice and develop social competence in their strategies for expressing resistance. We proposed that noncompliant behaviors could be viewed as the child's own strategies for persuading parents to drop or modify their requests and that, like parental discipline and control strategies, they vary in their sophistication and effectiveness. Some ways of saying "no" are more subtle and skilful than others.

A simple way of thinking about the categories is in terms of their directness and aversiveness for the parent. Of the active forms of noncompliance that we studied, direct defiance and whining sometimes accompanied by poorly controlled anger is likely to be perceived as both very direct and very aversive by parents. Simple refusals, an intermediate category in terms of skill, is direct but not as aversive. Finally, negotiation, attempts to persuade parents to modify their demands by active bargaining or explanation is relatively indirect and nonaversive as a social strategy. We considered negotiation to be a particularly sophisticated strategy because it is a way of saying "no" without actually saying "no".

Parents who might not tolerate direct opposition may accept children's attempts to negotiate as acceptable expressions of their autonomy and assertiveness.

Preliminary support for our developmental hypotheses were found in two studies: A cross-sectional study of children between the ages of 15 months and 51 months ((Kuczynski *et al.*, 1987) and a longitudinal study of the same children when they were followed up at age 5 years (Kuczynski & Kochanska, 1990). No age differences were found in children's compliance to their mothers' commands and prohibitions; what did change was the quality of their noncompliance. Direct defiance, the most obtrusive way of saying "no" as well as passive noncompliance decreased in frequency with age. In contrast, simple refusals and particularly, negotiation, increased with age of child.

Together, these findings indicate that as children develop during the toddler and preschool periods they are more likely to express their autonomy by actively resisting excessive control by their parents. However this developmental trend may not be an obvious one for all children because children also develop skills for expressing their autonomy in a socially appropriate manner. Our hypothesis is that children's negotiation strategies undergo further differentiation during childhood and gradually merge with what in an adult would be considered assertive socially competent behavior. A second hypothesis emerging from this developmental perspective is that an important component of the difficulty presented by children classed as oppositional and noncompliant in school age populations is that they display a level of skill in expressing their resistance that is more characteristic of much younger children.

The model of parental competence that emerges from this developmental model also diverges from that of the behavior modification perspective. We suspect that an important element in parental skill may be their ability to discriminate among different forms of noncompliance and to provide differential feedback for appropriate and inappropriate forms of resistance. At this point we have only indirect evidence that mothers discriminate between skilful and unskilful forms of noncompliance.(Kuczynski, *et al.*, 1989). First there is evidence that only unskilful forms of noncompliance are perceived as stressful by mothers. Correlations between toddler age children's responses to maternal control and minute by minute ratings of mother's negative affect observed during 6 hours of interactions with their children indicated that only unskilful forms of noncompliance, passive noncompliance and direct defiance, were positively related to mothers' negative affect. The relatively more skilful strategies of refusal and negotiation were not related to mother's negative affect.

Mothers' perceptions of their children's adjustment was also influenced by the quality of their children's opposition. Correlations between mothers' perceptions of behavior problems in their children (Achenbach & Edelbrock, 1981) and children's strategies for expressing noncompliance indicated that only the least skilful forms of resistance were predictive of children's behavior problems at age 5. Indeed, the toddler data suggested that children who assert their autonomy appropriately by means of simple refusals were less likely to be perceived as having behavior problems at age 5. A question for future research is whether parents actively promote children's learning of skilful ways of expressing their resistance to parental controls.

In summary, a rather complex model of children's obedience is required to understand the behavior of children and parents in child-rearing interactions. An underlying assumption of this model is that parents in well functioning families make some rather fine contextual discriminations that guide their efforts to secure their children's compliance and to appropriately respond to their children's noncompliance. However, even greater complexity needs to be incorporated into models of parental skill because cutting across each of the issues discussed in this chapter is the fact that parents also adapt their influence strategies to developmental changes occurring within their children. Attempts to systematically map the changes that occur in parent-child interactions during the course of children's development

(Kuczynski *et al.*, 1986; Kochanska, Kuczynski, & Maguire, 1989) and to understand the processes that underlie these changes (Dix & Grusec, 1983; Maccoby, 1984) are just beginning. But it is clear that something of the dynamic nature of socialization processes will be reflected in future conceptions of children's compliance and of parental competece.

References

Achenbach, T. M. & Edelbrock, C. S. (1981). Behavioral problems and competencies reported by parents of normal and disturbed children aged four through sixteen. *Monographs of the Society for Research in Child Development.* 46, No.1, Serial No. 188.

Baumrind, D. (1971). Current patterns of parental authority. *Developmental Psychology Monograph, 4*, (1, Pt 2).

Brehm, S.S. (1981). Oppositional behavior in children: A reactance theory approach. In S.S. Brehm, S.M. Kassin, F.K. Gibbons (Eds.), *Developmental Social Psychology: Theory and Research.* New York: Oxford Press.

Cheyne, J.A., & Walters, R.H. (1969). Intensity of punishment, timing of punishment, and cognitive structure as determinants of response inhibition. *Journal of Experimental Child Psychology*, 231-244.

Crockenberg, S. & Litman, C. (1987). Autonomy as competence in two-year-olds: Maternal correlates of child compliance, noncompliance and self-assertion. Paper presented at the Biennial Meetings of the Society for Research in Child Development in Baltimore.

Deci, E.L. & Ryan, R.M. (1987). The support of autonomy and the control of behavior. *Journal of Personality and Social Psychology.* 53, 1024-1037.

Dix, T.H. & Grusec, J.E. (1983). Parent attribution processes in child socialization. In I. Siegel (Ed.) *Parental Belief Systems: Their Psychological Consequences for Children.* Hillsdale, NJ: Lawrence Erlbaum Associates.

Eghrari, H. & Deci, E.L. (1986). *Facilitating Internalization: The role of self-determination.* Unpublished manuscript, University of Rochester. Rochester, New York.

Forehand, R. (1977). Child noncompliance to parental requests: Behavioral analysis and treatment. In M. Hersen, R.M. Eisler & P.M. Miller (eds). *Progress in Behavior Modification* (Volume 5). New York: Academic Press.

Forehand, R. L. and McMahon, R.J. (1981). *Helping the Noncompliant Child A Clinician's Guide to Parenting.* New York: The Guildford Press.

Grusec, J.E., & Kuczynski, L. (1980). Direction of effect in socialization: A comparison of parent versus child's behavior as determinants of disciplinary technique. *Developmental Psychology, 16*, 1-9.

Grusec, J.E. & Redler, E. (1980). Attribution, reinforcement, and altruism: A developmental analysis. *Developmental Psychology, 16*, 525-534.

Hetherington, E.M., Cox, M. & Cox, R. (1982). Effects of divorce on parents and children. In M. Lamb (Ed.), *Nontraditional Families.* Hillsdale, New Jersey: Lawrence Erlbaum Associates.

Hoffman, M.L. (1970). Moral Development. In P Mussen (Ed.) Carmichael's Manual of Child Psychology. Vol 2. New York: Wiley, 261-259.

Kochanska, G., Kuczynski, L. & Maguire, M. (1989). Impact of diagnosed depression and self-reported mood on mothers' control strategies. *Journal of Abnormal Child Psychology, 17*, 493-511.

Kopp, C.B. (1982). Antecedents of self-regulation: A developmental perspective. *Developmental Psychology, 18*, 199-214.

Kuczynski, L. (1982). Intensity and orientation of reasoning: Motivational determinants of children's compliance to verbal rationales. *Journal of Experimental Child Psychology, 34*, 357-370.

Kuczynski, L (1983). Reasoning, prohibitions and motivations for compliance. *Developmental Psychology, 19*, 126 -134.

Kuczynski, L. (1984). Socialization goals and mother-child interaction: Strategies for long-term and short-term compliance. *Developmental Psychology, 20*, 1061-1073.

Kuczynski, L., & Kochanska, G.(1990). The development of children's noncompliance strategies from toddlerhood to age 5. *Developmental Psychology, 26*, 398-408.

Kuczynski, L., Kochanska, G., Radke-Yarrow, M. & Girnius-Brown, O. (1987). A developmental interpretation of young children's noncompliance. *Developmental Psychology, 23*, 799-806.

Lay, K.L. & Waters, E.& Park, K.A. (1989). Maternal responsiveness and child compliance: The role of mood as a mediator. *Child Development, 60*, 1405-1411.

Leizer, J. I. & Rogers, R.W. (1974). Effects of method of discipline, timing of punishment, and timing of test on resistance to temptation. *Child Development, 45*, 790-793.

Lepper, M.R. (1973). Dissonance, self-perception, and honesty in children. *Journal of Personality and Social Psychology, 25*, 65-74.

Lepper, M.R. (1982). Social control processes, attributions of motivation, and the internalization of social values. In E.T. Higgins, D.N. Rubble, & W.W. Hartup (Eds.) *Social Cognition and Social Behavior: Developmental Perspectives*. Cambridge, England: Cambridge University Press.

Londerville, S., & Main, M. (1981). Security of attachment, compliance and maternal training methods in the second year of life. *Developmental Psychology, 17*, 289-299.

Longfellow, C., Zelkowitz, P. & Saunders, E. (1982). The quality of mother-child relationships. In D. Belle (ed.) *Lives in Stress*. London: Sage.

Lytton, H. (1980). *Parent-Child Interaction: The Socialization Process Observed in Twin and Singleton Families*. New York: Plenum.

Maccoby, E.E. (1984). Socialization and developmental change. *Child Development, 55*, 317-328.

Maccoby, E.E. & Martin,J.A. (1983). Socialization in the context of the family: Parent-child interaction. In E.M. Hetherington (Ed.) *Handbook of child psychology: Vol IV.Socialization,personality and social development*. New York: Wiley, (pp.1-101).

Martin, B. (1975). Parent-child relations. In F.D. Horowitz (Ed.) *Review of Child Development Research* (Vol. 4). Chicago: University of Chicago Press.

Matas,L., Arend, R., & Sroufe, L.(1978). Continuity of adaptation in the second year: The relationship between quality of attachment and later competence. *Child Development, 49,* 547-556.

Milgram, S. (1974). *Obedience to Authority: An Experimental View.* New York: Harper & Row.

Minton, C., Kagan, J. & Levine, J.A. (1971). Maternal control and obedience in the two year old. *Child Development, 42,* 1873-1894.

Newson, J. and Newson, E., (1968). *Four Years Old In An Urban Community.* Chicago: Aldine Publishing Co.

Parke, R.D. (1969). Effectiveness of punishment as an interaction of intensity, timing, agent nurturance and cognitive structuring. *Child Development, 40,* 231-236.

Parpal, M. & Maccoby, E.E. (1985). Maternal responsiveness and subsequent child compliance. *Child Development, 56,* 1326-1334.

Patterson, G.R. (1982). *Coercive Family Process.* Eugene, Oregon: Castillia Press.

Patterson, G & Forgatch, M.(1987). *Parents and Adolescents: Living Together.* Eugene, Oregon: Castalia Publishing Co.

Patterson, G. R. DeBarsyshe, B.D. & Ramsey, E. (1989) A developmental perspective on antisocial behavior. *American Psychologist, 44,* 329-335.

Patterson, G.R. (1986) Performance models for antisocial boys. *American Psychologist, 41,* 432-444.

Perry, D.G. & Perry, L.C. (1983). Social learning, causal attribution, and moral internalization. In J. Bisanz, G.L. Bisanz, & R. Kail (Eds.) *Learning in Children: Progress in Cognitive Development Research.* New York: Springer-Verlag, 105-136.

Reid, J.B. (1982). Social-Interactional Patterns in Families of Abused and Nonabused children. Paper presented at the Conference on Altruism and Aggression, Washington, D.C.in April.

Sears, R.R., Maccoby, E.E. & Levin, H. (1957). *Patterns of Child Rearing.* Evanston, Ill.: Row Peterson.

Stayton, D., Hogan, R. & Ainsworth, M.D.S. (1971). Infant obedience and material behavior: The origins of socialization reconsidered. *Child Development, 42,* 1057-1069.

Trickett, P.K. and Kuczynski, L. (1986). Children's misbehaviors and parental discipline strategies in abusive and nonabusive families. *Developmental Psychology, 22,* 115-123.

Vaughn, B.E., Kopp, C.B. & Krakow, J.B. (1984). The emergence and consolidation of self-control from eighteen to 30 months of age: Normative trends and individual differences. *Child Development, 55,* 990-1004.

Wenar, C. (1982). On negativism. *Human Development, 25,* 1-23.

Zahn-Waxler, C. Radke-Yarrow, M., & King, R..(1979). Childrearing and children's prosocial initiation towards victims of distress. *Child Development, 50,* 319-330.

Zelkowitz, P. (1982). Parenting philosophies and practices. In D. Belle (ed.) *Lives in Stress.* London: Sage.

A.J.E. de Veer & J.M.A.M. Janssens

Victim-Oriented Discipline and the Child's Internalization of Norms

An impressive body of research has grown up about the relationship between parental disciplinary techniques and a diversity of child outcome measures (Hoffman, 1970; Maccoby & Martin, 1983; Radke-Yarrow & Zahn-Waxler, 1986; Rollins & Thomas, 1979; Shaffer & Brody, 1981; Steinmetz, 1979). One of these child outcomes is moral development. In explaining the relation between discipline and moral development the role of the child's perspective taking ability is often mentioned (Hoffman, 1970; Maccoby & Martin, 1983). Studies indicate that the way parents react to their children is associated with the children's perspective taking ability (e.g., Peterson & Skevington, 1988; Silbereisen, 1976, 1977). In addition to these correlational studies, intervention efforts focusing on specific training of perspective taking skills has been shown to stimulate these skills (e.g., Chandler, 1973; Lowell Krogh, 1985). On the other hand, the hypothesized relation between perspective taking and moral development has also been investigated (e.g., Selman, 1971; Walker, 1980). The mediating role of perspective taking as an explanation of the influence of disciplinary techniques on moral development has not often been the focus of research. One of the exceptions is the chapter by Janssens and Gerris (this book) in which the mediating role of empathy in the relationship between discipline and prosocial development is explored. In this research we are interested in the influence of discipline on moral internalization. First, we explain why moral internalization depends on the child's capacity to take different perspectives. Second, we discuss how parents can promote the child's perspective taking ability.

Moral internalization will be defined in accord with Hoffman's formulation. Moral internalization means that the concern for others must be displayed independently of fear of punishment or hope of reward by external agents (Hoffman, 1975a). A child who has internalized norms, not only experiences hedonistic needs but is also motivated to take the needs of other persons into account. A child who has not yet internalized a moral norm is assumed to have a moral orientation based on fear of external detection and punishment. Hoffman (1970) used a subjective definition of external sanctions. External sanctions are not an objective feature but in the mind of the actor. A child can behave in accord with a moral standard in situations where detection is unlikely. But this behavior might be motivated by irrational fears of authority figures, or retribution by ghosts or gods. Moral internalization refers to a freedom from subjective concerns about external sanctions.

A moral norm is characterized by three components (Hoffman, 1983). First, the person feels an obligation to act in accord with the norm. Hoffman called this the affective and motivational component of a norm. Hoffman (1984a) asserted that affect, especially empathy, often functions as a motive for moral behavior. Empathy is defined as the affective response more appropriate to someone else's situation than to one's own (Hoffman, 1987). The activation of a moral norm does not guarantee moral action because the egoistic motive may be more powerful. Moral action is not simply the expression of a moral motive but the attempt to achieve an acceptable balance between one's egoistic and moral motives.

In addition to this affective-motivational component, moral norms also have a cognitive component which includes one's representation of the consequences that one's actual or anticipated behavior may have for someone else, one's awareness of prohibitions against acting in ways that may harm others physically or psychologically, and one's judgments about the rightness or wrongness of particular acts and the reasons for these judgments. These cognitions pertain to the shaping and transformations of the affective experience. When the child realizes that he/she has caused the observed distress (i.e. cognitive component) these feelings may be transformed into feelings of guilt.

The final component of moral internalization that Hoffman distinguished is the autonomous component. Activation of a moral norm is experienced as deriving autonomously from within the self. That is, the cognitive dimensions of a norm are thought of as one's own idea and the associated affect (usually guilt) and disposition to act in accord with the norm are experienced as coming from within the self.

To summarize, moral internalization refers to consideration of the needs of others and has a cognitive as well as a compelling, obligatory quality that is not based on fear of punishment. The internal motives are usually experienced as deriving from oneself. It seems obvious that the criterion of moral internalization is not whether or not certain information concerning norms is stored but the consideration of another's needs in subsequent moral encounters. In these new situations empathic arousal is seen as a motive for this consideration (Hoffman, 1982, 1987).

Which role does the child's perspective taking play in moral internalization? Perspective taking has been considered to be an important prerequisite of moral development (Kohlberg, 1976; Piaget, 1965; Selman, 1976; see also the chapter by Janssen, Janssens & Gerris). It is considered to be a necessary but not sufficient precondition to mature moral judgment (Kohlberg, 1976; Walker, 1980). The evidence for this relationship is equivocal. Several reviews of the empirical research found a lack of consistent relationships between perspective taking and variables such as prosocial behavior (Iannotti, 1985: Radke-Yarrow, Zahn-Waxler, & Chapman, 1983; Shantz, 1975, 1983), moral judgment, and altruism (Kurdek, 1978). In contrast, Underwood and Moore (1982) employed a meta-analytical technique to aggregate over independent studies and concluded that reliable relationships are to be found between perspective taking and altruism.

Hoffman (1983) also suggested that perspective taking is important to the internalization of moral norms, although this perspective has to be combined with empathic arousal. Infants are egocentric in the sense that they make no distinction between their view of social situations and possible alternative views. Older children may know that the other can hold a different perspective but they are unable to specify that perspective or they may merely assume similarity between their thoughts and the other's thoughts and intentions. During middle childhood children become able to infer the other's intentions, feelings and thoughts with a good deal of accuracy.

How does perspective taking relate to empathy? The child's ability to take the perspective of others may play a role in two ways. First, a child's initial affective reaction to another's distress may motivate the child to take the perspective of the other. Hoffman (1984a, 1987) assumed that a child has an inborn capacity to react affectively to the affect of another person. This affective response is influenced by the child's cognitive sense of the other. An infant is initially unable to distinguish between another's distress and one's own feelings of distress. However, when the child realizes, as a consequence of his or her perspective taking ability, that the experienced distress is a reaction to the other person's distress the child may become motivated to help the other person. When the child does not know the cause of his or her own feelings of distress he or she will not feel concern for the other person and, consequently, it is unlikely that the child would offer help. Thus the ability to understand the situation influences the child's subsequent behavior.

Second, an empathic reaction may be the consequence of taking another's perspective. Perspective taking involves understanding another's thoughts and motives as well as feelings. As the child becomes progressively better able to recognize the other is in need and to anticipate the consequences of his or her actions to others, the child feels empathy for the other person and is motivated to consider the needs of the other.

Thus, Hoffman assumed perspective taking is influenced by already present empathic feelings but may also elicit empathic feelings. These empathic feelings motivate the child to behave morally.

Hoffman (1975a, 1983, 1984b) suggested that disciplinary encounters within the family have a central role in stimulating moral internalization. In disciplinary encounters, the parent attempts to change the child's behavior. The child has done harm to another person, is going to harm someone, or omits helping another person who needs assistance. It appears as if the child either does not notice or neglects the needs of others. Whenever parents try to change the child's behavior they have to inform the child about their desire. This is what happens in a disciplinary encounter.

The parent may communicate that he or she disapproves of the child's behavior in many ways. Hoffman (1970) distinguished three categories of disciplinary techniques. Induction refers to techniques in which the parent gives explanations or reasons for requiring the child to change behavior (e.g., by pointing out the painful consequences of the child's behavior for others). A second category, power assertion, is defined as behavior of the parent which results in considerable external pressure on the child to behave according to the parent's desires. Power assertion includes physical punishment, deprivation of material objects or privileges, the direct application of force, or the threat of any of these. A third category of techniques, love withdrawal, is defined as nonphysical expression of the parent's anger or disapproval of the child with the implication that love will not be restored until the child changes his or her behavior (e.g., ignoring, isolating, or rejecting the child).

A child who receives a power assertive discipline probably has some idea (s)he has done something wrong. However, although power assertion may stimulate compliance, it is insufficient to promote internalization. In Hoffman's conceptualization of morality, internalization implies considering the needs of another. Because young children are hedonistically oriented and not aware of the needs of others, parents have to point out another's needs to the child.

However, before a child is able to process the information provided by the parent the child must be made to attend to the parent's message. Consequently, the discipline strategies actually used by parents are usually multidimensional (Hoffman, 1970, 1983). Most discipline reactions have power assertive (e.g., punishing, threatening) and love withdrawing (e.g., neglecting, isolating) properties which comprise the motive-arousal component needed to get the child to pay attention to the inductive component that may also be present. Too little arousal may prompt the child to ignore the parent. Too much arousal, producing fear, anxiety, or resentment, may prevent the effective processing of the inductive component and may direct the child's attention to the consequences of the action for the self. Inductive strategies can also arouse anxiety by means of the parent's tone of voice or the inherent message of disapproval which may threaten the child's feelings of security in the parent-child relationship. However, Hoffman suggested that an optimal level of arousal for processing information is more likely to be achieved by inductions (Hoffman, 1983a).

Research on child-rearing characteristics and moral internalization has been reviewed a number of times (e.g., Hoffman, 1963, 1970; Maccoby & Martin, 1983; Rollins & Thomas, 1979; Shaffer & Brody, 1981). Much research concerning the relation between disciplinary techniques used by the parent and the child's moral internalization was correlational, neglecting the causality problem and the variables which may mediate this relation. There is a lack of consistent relationship between inductive discipline and morality.

One possible explanation for the discrepant results is that parental variables can be defined and measured in several ways. Most studies defined induction as an undifferentiated category. Induction is a broad disciplinary category that includes many kinds of reasons and explanations. However, many studies suggest that there are qualitatively different categories of induction (Maccoby & Martin, 1983).

Hoffman (1970) singled out "other-oriented induction", that is, explanations that describe the implications of the child's behavior for other persons, as especially important to moral development. Hoffman and Saltzstein (1967) operationalized induction as messages referring to the consequences of the child's action for others. They differentiated between a category 'induction regarding parent' (e.g., the action has hurt the parent, that an object was valued by the parent) and 'induction regarding peers (e.g., the parent makes reference to and shows concern for the feelings of the victimized child). Induction regarding parents correlated more frequently with moral indices than induction regarding peers. In an attempt to explain the development of altruistic behavior, Hoffman (1975b) stressed the importance of 'victim-centered techniques'. These techniques include pointing up the harmful consequences of the child's behavior for the victim or asking the child to imagine him- or herself in the other person's place. However, unlike other-oriented induction, it also refers to techniques that suggest concrete acts of reparation and techniques that require the child to apologize.

Bearison and Cassel (1975) studied the effectiveness of verbal communication and differentiated between mothers making 'person-oriented statements' and mothers making 'position-oriented statements'. Person-oriented appeals include regulatory statements that draw attention to the feelings, thoughts, needs, or intentions of the mother, the child, or a third person who may be affected by the child's action. Position-oriented appeals refer to rules or statutes (e.g., "all children have to go to school"). They hypothesized that person-oriented statements are more effective because they stimulate the child to take the perspective of others. Children whose mothers used person-oriented arguments, rather than position-oriented ones, were more successful in taking the perspective of another person in a game that required them to do so.

In a study by Sims (cited in Keller & Bell, 1979) 'active induction' and 'passive induction' were differentiated. Active induction, a type in which the child actively participates by taking the other's role, was found to be more effective in stimulating altruistic behavior than passive induction (lecturing by the parent). This classification resembles the techniques of 'distancing' and of 'didactic induction' Peterson and Skevington (1988) used to investigate the relation between cognitive role-taking and child-rearing methods. Distancing typically involves questions that challenge the child's existing point of view, creating a cognitive conflict in the child. In operational terms didactic induction was defined as one-way communication strategies that provide logical reasons for the requested behavior change without encouraging the child to discover such reasons or to think spontaneously about their rationale. Distancing was significantly associated with the child's cognitive role-taking skills, but didactic induction was not related with role-taking skills.

Staub (1979) distinguished between 'positive induction' and 'negative induction'. He suggested that positive induction provided a stronger incentive value to act prosocially. Positive induction refers to pointing out the positive consequences of desirable behavior, the increased welfare of other people, the positive emotions that such behavior induces in the other person. Negative induction consists of pointing out the negative consequences of the child's undesirable behavior for other people.

Apparently, several types of induction can be distinguished which may have different effects on the child. Consequently, the correlation between the use of induction and the child's moral internalization can be suppressed when several types of induction are lumped all together.

We hypothesize that messages that direct the child's attention toward the victim are particularly likely to stimulate moral internalization because they promote the child's perspective taking. We use the term 'victim-oriented discipline'. Victim-oriented discipline directs the child's attention to the consequences of his or her behavior for someone else rather than for the self (e.g., "Look, now he is sad because you took his favorite toy"), teaches the child to refrain from moral transgressions (e.g., "How do you think X will feel if you break his toy"), and teaches the child to help another (e.g., "Make up to the child for what you have done"). As a result the child can make a causal connection between his or her own action and the physical or psychological state of the victim.

The goal of the present study was twofold. The relationship between victim-oriented discipline and moral internalization was investigated. Furthermore we examined the mediating role of perspective taking skills. Parents favoring victim-oriented discipline were predicted to have children with advanced perspective taking skills and, consequently, with advanced moral internalization.

Method

Subjects
The sample consisted of 150 families with a child attending the second, fourth, or sixth grade, randomly selected from fourteen elementary schools in the neighborhood of Nijmegen, a town of 140,000 inhabitants in the east of the Netherlands. At least one parent of each child participated. The total sample consisted of 150 mothers, 132 fathers, 72 boys and 78 girls. Forty-seven children attended second grade (23 boys, 24 girls, $M = 5;9$ years), 50 children attended fourth grade (24 boys, 26 girls, $M = 7;11$ years), and 53 children attended sixth grade (25 boys, 28 girls, $M = 9;10$ years).

Ninety-three percent of the families were two-parent families. The occupational status of the fathers was classified on the basis of 'I.T.S. Beroepenklapper' (Westerlaak van, Kropman & Collaris, 1975). Three percent of the fathers was classified as unskilled labourers, 21% skilled labourers, 20% low level employees, 9% self-employed persons, 19% mid level employees, and 21% higher occupation. There was an underrepresentation of the two lower levels and an overrepresentation of the two top levels.

Measurement
Parental victim-oriented discipline
Parental discipline was assessed by interviewing each parent. Each respondent was asked to react to nine hypothetical situations. In each situation the son or daughter transgressed or intended to transgress a norm by victimizing another child. Because situational characteristics, such as intention of the child and the consequences of the transgression, influence the parental disciplinary reaction (Grusec & Kuczynski, 1980; Janssens, Janssen, Bernaerts & Gerris, 1985) the situations varied on these aspects. One of the stories was:
Your son and his friend are playing. Suddenly, your son tears the new shirt of his friend. The friend looks dismayed.
Following each situation the parents were asked how they would react in such situation. The situations were presented in random order.

The reaction of the parent to each hypothetical situation was coded with a modified version of the coding system used by Grusec and Kuczynski (1980). The coding system listed 27 disciplinary practices (inter-rater reliability was 77%) such as physical punishment, deprivation of material objects or priviliges, ignoring the child, disapproval of the child's behavior, suggesting alternative ways of behaving, referring to the consequences of the child's action for the victim, and stimulating to repair the damage. The general category 'victim-oriented discipline' consisted of behavior categories stressing the position of the victim, i.e. referring to the material and/or personal consequences of the child's action for the victim and stimulating to repair the damage and/or to apologize. If the parent uses many types of disciplinary strategies in response to the same misbehavior the victim-oriented message may be diffused. Other disciplinary reactions may distract the child's attention from the victim. Consequently, in every situation the impact of victim-oriented discipline was related to the total number of disciplinary reactions. These nine proportions were averaged to obtain the parent's score on victim-oriented discipline.

Perspective taking
The development in perspective taking has been operationalized by Selman as a progressive increase in the number of elements and relations that must be kept in mind (Higgins, 1981). Selman (1976) distinguished several domains in which the level of perspective taking is manifested. In this research we confined ourselves to the domain of parent-child relations. Several questions about parent-child relationship were asked. The questions referred to four characteristic issues of the parent-child relationship: function and rationale for punishment (e.g., "Why do parents sometimes punish their children?", "Do you think that children should be punished when they disobey?", "How does punishment work?", "What does it do for children?"), demands for obedience (e.g., "Should children always obey their parents?", "Why do parents want their children to obey them?"), factors that cause conflicts (e.g., "What are some of the reasons that parents and children do not get along?"), and methods parents and children have for conflict resolution (e.g., "How can you best end a disagreement?").

The child's perspective on every issue was scored according to the system developed by Bruss-Saunders (Selman, 1979). At the lowest level (stage 0) the child has egocentric and pragmatic conceptions of the parent-child relationship. Stage 1 conceptions are characterized by an identification with parental views. The main characteristic of stage 2 conceptions is their focus on the quality of the emotional ties between parent and child. And at the highest level coded in this investigation (stage 3) the parent-child relationship is considered to be both a reflection of and influence on the parent's and the child's personality functioning. The four scores were averaged together into a mean issue score (Selman, 1979). Inter-rater reliabilities were 79% for function and rationale for punishment, 78% for demands for obedience, and 79% and 83% for causes and resolutions of conflicts respectively.

Moral internalization

Several moral indices were used, each tapping a different aspect of moral internalization. Hoffman distinguished four indicators of moral internalization (Hoffman, 1970; Hoffman & Saltzstein, 1967): (1) the use of moral judgments about others which are based on internal rather than external considerations; (2) the intensity of guilt experienced following own transgressions; (3) whether the child confesses and accepts responsibility for own misdeeds; (4) the degree to which the child can be counted on to resist pressures to deviate even when the possibility of detection and punishment are remote.

To assess these indicators we interviewed the children and we asked the teacher of each child to complete a questionnaire. Children were administered the Socio-Moral Interview (S.M.I., Veer de, Janssens & Gerris, 1987). The S.M.I. consists of four hypothetical stories describing a socio-moral situation. Each story concerns a child who transgresses a norm (taking away a child's toy, hurting someone, deceiving someone, breaking another's toy). The protagonist in the stories is of the same sex and same age as the child. The interviewer read each story to the child and demonstrated each story with pictures. An example of the stories is:

> This child is playing with his new ball. The ball rolls into the road and a car runs over the ball. The ball is broken. The child sadly walks away. The child then sees his friend playing with a ball and starts crying. He then snatches the ball on purpose. Now his friend doesn't have a ball and starts to cry.

After checking whether a child understood each story, a set of standardized questions was asked. This set of questions was repeated after each story. Both stories and the questions within each set were presented in random order. A short version of the S.M.I. (two stories) was conducted with the youngest age group because of the attentional limited capacity.[1]

---

1. It was possible that the two stories of the short version of the S.M.I. revealed different answers when compared with the two extra stories in the original S.M.I.. This would make it difficult to compare the answers of the second grade children with the other children. To investigate possible differences

The four indicators of moral internalization were:

1. *Internalized moral judgments*. The child was asked to judge the transgression in the S.M.I.-story (e.g., "Are you allowed to snatch toys of other children?", "Why?/Why not?"). In each story the child's response was coded as external (score 0, e.g., "you will be punished"), internal (score 2, e.g., "you will hurt another child, it will make him sad"), or indeterminate (score 1). Inter-rater reliability was 88%. The mean score of all stories was computed and constituted the child's internalization score of moral judgment.

2. *Guilt*. Guilt is defined as a conscious self-initiated and self-critical reaction to transgression (Hoffman, 1970). Two (projective) guilt measures, analogous to the guilt measures of Thompson and Hoffman (1980), were used to assess guilt:

   Concern for victim. The child was encouraged to identify with the transgressor of the S.M.I.-story. Subsequently, the child was asked to express the post-transgression feelings of the transgressor with whom the child identified. The children were also asked to provide an ending to the story. The guilt measure was based on the child's explicit expressions of concern for the victim (in contrast to self-concern, such as worry over detection). The answers were coded on a three-point scale (inter-rater reliability was 80%). No guilt feelings or feelings based on self-concern were scored as 0. Feelings based on a violation of conventional principles were scored as 1. Explicit expressions of concern for the victim were scored as 2. The child's guilt response as expressed in concern for the victim was obtained by averaging the scores of concern for the victim.

   Use of justice principles. A second guilt measure was based on the quality of justice principles offered to explain guilt feelings. The children were asked whether they would feel differently if the act remained undetected by others. The measure was coded on a three-point scale (inter-rater reliability was 80%). Expressions of self-concern were scored as 0. Answers expressing justice principles such as mutual thrust or personal rights were coded as 2. Answers which on the one hand contained principles of justice but on the other hand expressed relief when the act remained undetected

---

between the two sets of stories we averaged the scores at the first story-pair and the scores at the second story-pair for every variable and each fourth and sixth grade child. T-tests revealed no significant differences between the average scores ($p > .05$) of the two story-pairs.

were coded as 1. The child's guilt response as expressed in the use of justice principles was obtained by averaging the scores of use of justice principles.

3. *Resistance to deviation.* The strength of children's resistance to deviate from a norm was operationalized in a subscale of the teacher questionnaire. The subscale consisted of three items, e.g., "I have to keep an eye on him to prevent him to do something wrong". The frequency of this behavior was scored on a six-point scale).

4. *Willingness to confess and accept responsibility.* Another four-item subscale of the teacher questionnaire assessed willingness to confess and accept responsibility when the child has done something wrong (e.g., "He shows guilt after wrongdoing", "He tries to repair after wrongdoing"). Because the subscales resistance to deviation and willingness to confess and accept responsibility were strongly correlated ($r = .52$, $p < .001$), the items were combined into one scale "moral behavior" (7 items, alpha = .86).

Analysis

In this study we analyzed relations between victim-oriented discipline (maternal and parental), perspective taking and moral internalization. Perspective taking and moral internalization are positively related to children's age. Some authors assumed that victim-oriented discipline also relates to children's age: parents react more inductively when an older child transgresses than when a younger child does, because an older child would understand the inductive message better than a younger child (Saltzstein, 1976). Because of the possibility that all correlations could be spurious due to the child's age, we analyzed the relations between victim-oriented discipline, perspective taking and moral internalization using partial correlations (with child's age being partialled out).

The main aim of this study was to test a model (Figure 1) describing how the influence of maternal and paternal victim-oriented discipline on moral internalization is mediated by perspective taking.

We tested the model with LISREL-analysis (Jöreskog & Sörbom, 1981). In this analysis relations between various theoretical constructs are examined. Each construct is called a latent factor and consists of one or more variables. If the four measures of moral internalization are related to each other, we can construct one latent factor (moral internalization) with loadings of the measured variables internalized

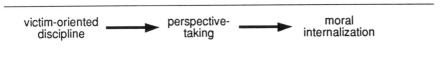

Figure 1   The hypothesized model

moral judgment, concern for the victim, use of justice principles, and moral behavior. Besides this latent factor there are three other latent factors in the LISREL-model, perspective taking, and maternal and paternal victim-oriented discipline. Each of these factors consists of only one measured variable, the average score of perspective taking and the proportion of maternal and paternal victim-oriented discipline respectively.

Results

In Table 1 partial correlations between victim-oriented discipline and perspective taking and several measures of moral internalization are presented.

Paternal victim-oriented discipline was not related to any measure of moral internalization. Maternal victim-oriented discipline was positively related to three of the four measures of moral internalization. Children of inductive mothers were more concerned about the victim, used more justice principles and more internalized moral judgments than children whose mothers reacted less inductive on transgressions. There was however no relation between maternal victim-oriented discipline and moral behavior. Maternal and paternal victim-oriented discipline were both positively related to perspective taking. The more the parent stressed the position of the victim the higher the capacity of the child to take the perspective of others.

In Table 2 partial correlations between perspective taking and several measures of moral internalization are presented. All relations between perspective taking and the four measures of moral internalization were statistically significant. The higher the level of perspective taking, the higher the level of moral internalization. Second, three measures of moral internalization (concern for the victim, use of justice principles and use of internalized moral judgments) were positively related to each other, but not related to moral behavior.

Because of this finding it was not possible to test the model presented in Figure 1. In Figure 1 moral internalization is represented

Table 1   Partial Correlations Between Victim-Oriented Discipline,
          Perspective Taking and Moral Internalization (with Child's Age
          partialled out)

| | Victim-oriented discipline | |
	mother	father
Perspective taking	.19*	.15*
Moral internalization		
– concern for victim	.16*	.04
– use of justice principles	.21*	.10
– use of internalized moral judgments	.16*	.05
– moral behavior	.03	.01

* $p < 0.05$

Table 2   Partial Correlations Between the Measures of Perspective Taking
          and Moral Internalization (with Child's Age partialled out)

| | Perspective taking | Moral internalization | | |
| | | concern for victim | justice principles | internalized judgments |
Moral internalization:				
concern for victim	.19*			
justice principles	.34*	.61*		
internalized judgments	.24*	.29*	.26*	
moral behavior	.19*	-.01	.09	.13

* $p < 0.05$

by one latent factor but results showed that the indicator of moral
behavior was not related to the three other aspects of moral internalization. Therefore we decided to construct two latent factors: moral

behavior and guilt. The first factor consisted only of the variable moral behavior and the second factor consisted of the other three measures of moral internalization: concern for the victim, use of justice principles and use of internalized moral judgments. The first two measures are indicators of guilt (Hoffman, 1970). Children scoring high on concern for the victim and use of justice principles are assumed to feel guilty and refer to the distress and rights of the victim. An internalized moral jugdment can also be considered as an indicator af guilt. A child who refers to the distress of a potential victim when asked why an act is wrong shows an internalized judgment. Thus a child who refers to the distress of the (potential) victim displays a concern for the victim, use of justice principles (e.g., fairness, rights of another), as well as an internalized moral judgment. On the other hand, children who frequently refer to external sanctions and authority figures always have low scores on these three indicators. Therefore, it was not surprising that these indicators loaded on one factor.

Besides these latent factors of moral behavior and guilt, we had two latent factors for victim-oriented discipline: maternal and parental discipline and one latent factor for perspective taking in the LISREL-analysis. For latent factors with only one measured indicator, the loading of this indicator was set equal to one. That means that the latent factor is identical with the variable of the same name. This was the case for the latent factors maternal and paternal victim-oriented discipline, perspective taking, and moral behavior. In the LISREL-analysis loadings of the three measured variables (concern for victim, use of justice principles, and internalized moral judgment) on the latent factor guilt were estimated as well as the effect of latent factors on the other latent factors. In our model we estimated the effect of maternal and paternal victim-oriented discipline on perspective taking and the influence of perspective taking on moral behavior and guilt. The results of the Lisrel-analysis are presented in Figure 2.

The Figure shows loadings of the variables (the rectangular forms) on the latent factors (the oval forms) and standardized regression-coefficients (the coefficients on the arrows between latent factors). The overall fit of the model was acceptable (chi-square=12.36, d.f.=12, p=.417). All hypothesized factor loadings and all regression coefficients but one were statistically significant ($p < .05$). The influence of paternal discipline on perspective taking was nearly significant ($p < .10$). We concluded that perspective taking has a positive influence on guilt and moral behavior and that perspective taking is influenced by maternal victim-oriented discipline. Therefore, perspective taking can be seen as mediating between maternal victim-oriented discipline and the child's moral internalization. Besides the indirect effect of maternal discipline on guilt there was also a direct effect. That means the influence of maternal discipline on guilt is not only mediated by perspective taking but also by other processes or variables.

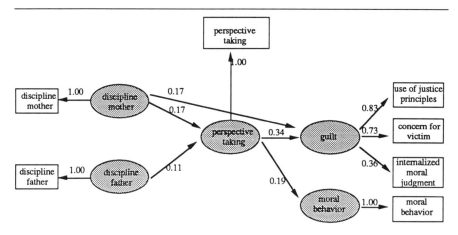

Chi-square = 12.36, d.f. = 12, p = .417.
The regression coefficient of victim-oriented discipline father to perspective taking is not significant.

Figure 2 The model tested by Lisrel analysis

Discussion

Dimensions of morality are sometimes treated as indices of a single underlying construct of 'moral development'. Results indicated that moral development is not a unitary construct. The four aspects of morality reflected two, independent, dimensions. These dimensions we called 'guilt' and 'moral behavior'. The 'guilt' dimension was considered as a latent factor indicated by three measures of moral internalization: concern for the victim, use of justice principles, and an internalized moral judgment. Thompson and Hoffman (1980) regarded a concern for the victim and the use of justice principles, which underlies feelings of remorse, as indicators of guilt experience. Consequently, when operationalizing the concept guilt, we not only asked the children to indicate the intensity of feelings of remorse they expected to experience after transgression, but also asked for the rationale of the reported feelings and whether their feelings would change when the act went undetected. Children with high scores on concern for the victim and use of justice principles did not worry about external punishment but emphasized the distress of the victim or the importance of mutual trust or personal rights. As a result the latent factor 'guilt' consisted of an affective component (the experienced feelings of remorse after transgression) and a cognitive component (the rationale for these feelings). The latent factor was also indicated by the child's use of internalized moral judgments. However, the loading of this variable was moderate. Most probably this was because moral judgments only assessed a cognitive aspect of morality: why a particular act is allowed or not allowed. The child's answers may refer to the distress of others caused by such an act or to more universal values as trust or personal rights. These answers resemble the answers children can give in response to the questions about their guilt experiences (concern for the victim and the use of justice principles). Therefore it is not surprising that the use of internalized moral judgments had a loading on the latent factor 'guilt'.

A second dimension of internalization was moral behavior. The scope of behaviors within this dimension was limited to the child's behavior in the classroom reported by the teacher. It is possible that moral behavior is situation-specific and thus the child may act differently in the classroom than outside the classroom. In particular, the child may be motivated to behave morally in the classroom but not in other situations. Furthermore we must take into account problems of validity associated with this behavioral measure. Teachers were asked to indicate the degree of resistance to deviation and willingness to confess after transgression demonstrated by the child. The occurrence of such behaviors does not necessarily reflect the internalization of norms. The manifestation of this behavior may also represent compliance or the seeking of social approval.

The LISREL-analysis showed no relation between guilt and moral behavior. Other authors have already indicated that moral judgments or feelings are not always expressed in behavior (e.g., Blasi, 1980; Eisenberg, 1982; Eisenberg, Shell, Pasternack, Lennon, Beller & Mathy, 1987; Radke-Yarrow, Zahn-Waxler & Chapman, 1983). According to Maccoby (1980), in concrete situations a number of implications of the act are considered (e.g., other's needs, self-interest, available information about the situation, the presence of other persons). These considerations can cause a discrepancy between judgment and actual behavior.

Our findings suggest that parental discipline is related to children's moral development. In particular, maternal victim-oriented discipline was positively related to guilt. However, no relation was found between maternal discipline and moral behavior. A possible explanation is the lack of an association between guilt and moral behavior. Mothers may influence the development of guilt through a guilt inducing discipline technique such as victim-oriented discipline. However, they cannot guarantee the transference from guilt experience into moral behavior. A second possible explanation is that we measured compliance rather than morally motivated behavior. There seems to be a relation between compliance and the use of power assertion (Saltzstein, 1976). Power assertion can compel the child to end the undesired behavior or to avoid this behavior. Power assertion can also stimulate the child to make reparations. However, if the behavior was perceived as being externally forced by some children, than we may have measured compliance and not internalization of these children. Therefore, the hypothesized relation between induction and moral behavior needs not to be found.

Only maternal victim-oriented discipline was positively related to the child's moral internalization (guilt). No relations were found between paternal discipline and guilt. This pattern is consistent with Hoffman's conclusion (1970) that an advanced moral orientation is associated with the mother's frequent use of inductive discipline. Also in Hoffman's studies very few relations were found between father's practices and the child's moral development (Hoffman, 1970). According to Hoffman (1975b) the role of the mother as a primary caretaker and the frequent absence or low level of involvement of the father may account for the lack of relations between paternal discipline and child variables. In our sample many mothers were the primary caretakers. Ninety-five percent of the fathers and thirty-one percent of the mothers in our sample had jobs outside the home. However, all but one of these fathers worked more than thirty hours a week and only six mothers worked more than thirty hours a week.

Victim-oriented discipline was found to have an indirect and a direct effect on guilt. The findings support the hypothesis that perspective taking mediates between maternal victim-oriented discipline and guilt. Victim-oriented discipline, operationalized as stressing the consequences of another and stimulating reparations, may have various consequences. It may increase children's ability to infer other's emotions and thus will increase their sensitivity for others. By pointing out the needs of the other person a parent may create a conflict between hedonistic needs and the needs of others. This conflict is an important aspect of moral internalization (Hoffman, 1975a). Victim-oriented discipline was distinguished from inductive messages or one-way communication strategies which give explanations and reasons. For example, "If everyone did this the world would be a mess", "If you act like this you will loose all your friends". Peterson and Skevington (1988) called this didactic induction. Some parents only used explanations without challenging the child's existing point of view or stimulating the child to rectify. These disciplinary reactions may not direct the child's attention to other's distress and may not explain the nature of it. Victim-oriented discipline, however, directs the child's attention to other's distress which may stimulate the child's perspective taking and as a consequence the development of guilt experiences.

Victim-oriented discipline also directly influenced guilt. This influence was not mediated by the child's capacity to take perspectives. Other processes or variables should be responsible for this effect. In our opinion perspective taking primarily influences the cognitive aspects of the guilt dimension. As mentioned above our guilt-concept combined an affective and a cognitive component. The child was asked to indicate feelings of remorse after transgression and also to reflect upon these feelings. When the child stressed the distress and the situation of the other, the child showed the perspective taking capacity. But a high guilt score depended not only on the content of the rationale but also on the presence of feelings of guilt. These feelings are not necessarily a consequence of the child's perspective taking. Guilt feelings can be caused by feelings of empathy or sympathy (Hoffman, 1987). Furthermore, inductive discipline was found to correlate positively with feelings of empathy and sympathy (Fultz, Batson, Fortenbach, McCarthy & Varney, 1986; Howard & Barnett, 1981; Toi & Batson, 1982; see chapter by Janssens & Gerris). According to Hoffman and Saltzstein (1967), induction motivates children to focus their attention on the harm done to another as the salient aspect of their transgression and thus helps to integrate their capacity for empathy with the knowledge of the consequences of their behavior. Therefore perspective taking is not necessarily the only possible mediator of victim-oriented discipline and guilt. Empathic and/or sympathetic feelings may also mediate this relation.

Another possible explanation of the direct influence of victim-oriented discipline on guilt is that victim-oriented discipline can be considered as one element of a larger child-rearing pattern. Inductive discipline is often combined with support and demandingness (Dekovic, Gerris & Janssens, 1991). Mothers who are inductive are often also more supportive and more demanding. Support is behavior manifested by a parent toward a child that makes the child feel confortable in the presence of the parent and confirms in the child's mind that he or she is basically accepted and approved as a person by the parent (Rollins & Thomas, 1979). Demandingness is behavior by which the parent makes an appeal to the child's responsibility, to mature behavior, to independence or to resolution of problems. Relations are found between support and moral development (Hoffman & Saltzstein, 1967; Rollins & Thomas, 1979; Staub, 1979) and between demandingness and moral development (Maccoby, 1980). According to Staub (1979) support makes the child feel secure and would minimize self-concern. Second, a supportive relationship with parents is likely to create a positive orientation toward other people. Concern about others' well-being may be promoted by support. A third consequence of support may be that it facilitates learning in the child, both in general and with regard to norms. Finally, support may be an important source of identification with parents. If the parent holds similar moral values the supportive relation with the parent would contribute to the acquisition of a moral orientation through identification.

Victim-oriented discipline is also related to demandingness. When parents are demanding they make an appeal to the child's responsibility. The same holds for victim-oriented discipline. It communicates to children that they are responsible for the distress of another person. If parents demand that their children have to consider the needs of others or if they teach that their children are responsible to help another they might promote their children's empathic capacities and therefore moral development.

A final comment has to be made about the direction of influences in this research. We looked only for evidence of parental influence on their children. This does not exclude the possibility that the child's moral intenalization influences the way parents discipline. Saltzstein (1976) proposed a model which shows that moral internalization can influence parental discipline. He suggested that moral development of children may determine the social influences to which they are suspectible, which in turn shape the kind of discipline the parents will use. However, our research focused on the influence of parental discipline on morality and the mediating role of perspective taking. Our findings were consistent with this one-directional model.

References

Bearison, D., & Cassel, T. (1975). Cognitive decentration and social codes: communicative effectiveness in young children from differing family contexts. *Developmental Psychology, 11,* 29-36.

Bell, R. (1968). A reinterpretation of the direction of effect in studies of socialization. *Psychological Review, 75,* 81-95.

Blasi, A. (1980). Bridging moral cognition and moral action: a critical review of the literature. *Psychological Bulletin, 88,* 1-45.

Chandler, M. (1973). Egocentrism and antisocial behavior. The assessment and training of social perspective-taking skills. *Developmental Psychology, 9,* 326-332.

Dekovic, M., Gerris, J., & Janssens, J. (1990). Parental cognitions, Parental behavior, and the child's understanding of parent – child relationship. *Merrill-Palmer Quarterly, 37,* 523-541.

Eisenberg, N. (1982). *The development of prosocial behavior.* New York: Academic Press.

Eisenberg, N., Shell, R., Pasternack, J., Lennon, R., Beller, R, & Mathy (1987). Prosocial development in middle childhood: A longitudinal study. *Developmental Psychology, 23,* 712-718.

Fultz, J., Batson, C., Fortenbach, V., McCarthy, P., & Varney, L. (1986). Social evaluation and the empathy-altruism hypothesis. *Journal of Personality and Social Psychology, 50,* 761-769.

Grusec, J. E., & Kuczynski, L. (1980). Direction of effect in socialization. A comparison of the parent's versus the child's behavior as determinants of disciplinary techniques. *Developmental Psychology, 16,* 1-19.

Higgins, E. T. (1981). Role taking and social judgment: alternative developmental perspectives and processes. In J. H. Flavell, & L. Ross (eds.), *Social cognitive development: Frontiers and possible futures* (pp. 119-153). Cambridge: Cambridge University Press.

Hoffman, M. L. (1963). Child rearing practices and moral development: generalizations from empirical reseach. *Child Development, 34,* 295-318.

Hoffman, M. L. (1970). Moral Development. In H.P. Mussen (ed.), *Carmichael's Handbook of Child Psychology* : Vol. II. (pp. 261-359). New York: Wiley.

Hoffman, M. L. (1975a). Moral internalization, parental power, and the nature of parent-child interaction. *Developmental Psychology, 11,* 228-239.

Hoffman, M. L. (1975b). Altruistic behavior and the parent-child relationship. *Journal of personality and social psychology, 31,* 937-943.

Hoffman, M. L. (1982). Development of prosocial motivation: empathy and guilt. In N. Eisenberg (ed), *The development of prosocial behavior* (pp.281-313). New York: Academic Press.

Hoffman, M. L. (1983). Affective and cognitive processes in moral internalization. In E. T. Higgins, D. N. Ruble, & W. W. Hartup (eds.), *Social cognition and social development. A socio-cultural perspective* (pp. 235-265). Braunschweig: Agentur Pedersen.

Hoffman, M. L. (1984a). Interaction of affect and cognition in empathy. In C. E. Izard, J. Kagan, & R. B. Zajonc (eds.), *Emotions, cognition and behavior* (pp. 103-131). Cambridge: Cambridge University Press.

Hoffman, M. L. (1984b). Parent discipline, moral internalization and development of prosocial motivation. In E. Staub, D. Bar-Tal, J. Karylowski, & J. Reykowski (eds.), *Development and maintenance of prosocial behavior* (pp. 117-137). New York: Plenum Press.

Hoffman, M. L. (1987). The contribution of empathy to justice and moral judgment. In N. Eisenberg, & J. Strayer (eds.), *Empathy and its development* (pp. 47-80). Cambridge: Cambridge University Press.

Hoffman, M. L., & Saltzstein, H. D. (1967). Parent discipline, and the child's moral development. *Journal of personality and social psychology, 5*, 45-57.

Howard, J., & Barnett, M. (1981). Arousal of empathy and subsequent generosity in young children. *Journal of Genetic Psychology, 138*, 307-308.

Iannotti, R. J. (1985). Naturalistic and structured assessments of prosocial behavior in preschool children: the influence of empathy and perspective taking. *Developmental Psychology, 21*, 46-54.

Janssens, J., Janssen, J., Bernaerts, M., & Gerris, J. (1985). *Disciplinering en situationale kenmerken*. Nijmegen: KUN, Empirische Pedagogiek.

Jöreskog, K. G., & Sörbom, D. (1981). *LISREL V: Analysis of linear structural relationships by maximum likelihood and least squares methods*. Chicago.

Keller, B. B., & Bell, R. Q. (1979). Child effects on adult's method of eliciting altruistic behavior. *Child Development, 50*, 1004-1009.

Kohlberg, L. (1976). Moral stages and moralisation. The cognitive-developmental approach. In T. Lickona (ed.), *Moral Development and behavior .Theory, research and social issues* (pp.253-265). New York: Holt, Rinehart, & Winston.

Kurdek, L. A. (1978). Perspective-taking as the cognitive basis of children's moral development: A review of the literature. *Merrill-Palmer Quarterly, 24*, 3-28.

Lowell Krogh, S. (1985). Encouraging positive justice reasoning and perspective-taking skills: two educational interventions. *Journal of moral education, 14*, 102-110.

Maccoby, E. (1980). *Social development: Psychological growth and the parent-child relationship*. New York: Harcourt Brace Jonavovich.

Maccoby, E.E., & Martin, J. A. (1983). Socialization in the context of the family: parent-child interaction. In H.P. Mussen (ed.), *Carmichael's Handbook of Child Psychology : Vol. IV. Socialization, personality and social development* (pp. 1-101). New York: Wiley.

Peterson, C., & Skevington, S. (1988). The relation between young children's cognitive role-taking and mothers' preference for a conflict-inducing childrearing method. *Journal of Genetic Psychology, 149*, 163-174.

Piaget, J. (1965). *The moral judgement of the child*. London: Routledge and Kegan Paul.

Radke-Yarrow, M., & Zahn-Waxler, C. (1986). The role of familial factors in the development of prosocial behavior: research findings and questions. In D. Olweus, J. Block, & M. Radke-Yarrow (eds.), *Development of antisocial and prosocial behavior. Research, theories, and issues* (pp.207-233). London: Academic Press.

Radke-Yarrow, M., Zahn-Waxler, C., & Chapman, M. (1983). Children's prosocial dispositions and behavior. In E. M. Hetherington (ed.), *Handbook of child psychology: Vol IV. Socialization, personality, and social development* (pp. 469-546). New York: Wiley.

Rollins, B. C., & Thomas, D. L. (1979). Parental support, power and control techniques in the socialization of children. In W. R. Burr, R. Hill, F. I. Nye, & I. L. Reiss (eds.), *Contemporary theories about the family: Vol. 1. Research based theories* (pp. 317-364). London: Free Press.

Saltzstein, H. D. (1976). Social influence and moral development. A perspective on the role of parents and peers. In T. Lickona (ed), *Moral development and behavior. Theory, research and social issues* (pp. 253-265). New York: Holt, Rinehart, & Winston.

Selman, R. L. (1971). Taking another's perspective: role-taking development in early childhood. *Child Development, 42*, 1721-1734.

Selman, R. L. (1976). Social-cognitive Understanding. A guide to educational and clinical practice. In T. Lickona (ed), *Moral development and behavior. Theory, research and social issues* (pp. 299-316). New York: Holt, Rinehart, & Winston.

Selman, R. L. (1979). *Assessing interpersonal understanding: an interview and scoring manual in five parts constructed by the Harvard-Judge Baker Social Reasoning Project.* Boston: Judge Baker Guidance Center.

Shaffer, D., & Brody, G. (1981). Parental and peer influences on moral development. In R. W. Henderson (ed.), *Parent-child interaction. Theory, research and prospects* (pp. 83-124). New York: Academic Press.

Shantz, C. (1975). The development of social cognition. In E. M. Hetherington (ed.), *Review of child development research: Vol V* (pp. 257-324). Chicago: University of Chicago Press.

Shantz, C. (1983). Social cognition. In P. H. Mussen, & E. M. Hetherington (eds.), *Handbook of child psychology: Vol IV. Social Development* (pp. 495-550). New York: Wiley.

Silbereisen, R. (1976). Prinzipierte mütterliche Erziehungseinstellungen und Rollenübernahme bei Kindern. *Zeitschrift für Entwicklungspsychologie und Pädagogische Psychologie, 8*, 288-297.

Silbereisen, R. (1977). Prädiktoren der Rollenübernahme bei Kinder. *Psychologie in Erziehung und Unterricht, 24*, 86-92.

Staub, E. (1979). *Positive social behavior and morality: socialization and development (vol. 2).* New York: Academic Press.

Steinmetz, S. K. (1979). Disciplinary techniques and their relationship to aggressivenes, dependency, and conscience. In W. Burr, R. Hill, F. Nye, & I. Reiss (eds.), *Contemporary theories about the family: Vol. 1. Research based theories* (pp. 405-438). London: Free Press.

Thompson, R., & Hoffman, M. (1980). Empathy and the development of guilt in children. *Developmental Psychology, 16,* 155-156.

Toi, M., & Batson, C. (1982). More evidence that empathy is a source of altruistic motivation. *Journal of personality and social psychology, 43,* 281-292.

Underwood, B., & Moore, B. (1982). Perspective taking and altruism. *Psychological Bulletin, 91,* 143-173.

Veer, A. de, Janssens, J., & Gerris, J. (1987). *Het Socio-Moreel Interview.* Nijmegen: KUN, Empirische Pedagogiek.

Walker, L. J. (1980). Cognitive and perspective-taking prerequisites for moral development. *Child Development, 51,* 131-139.

Westerlaak, J. M. van, Kropman, J. A., & Collaris, J. W. (1975). *Beroepenklapper.* Nijmegen: Instituut voor Toegepaste Sociologie.

Yarrow, M. R., Waxler, C., & Scott, P. (1971). Child effects on adult behavior. *Developmental Psychology, 5,* 300-311.

A.W.H. Janssen, J.M.A.M. Janssens, J.R.M. Gerris

Parents' and Children's Levels of Moral Reasoning: Antecedents and Consequences of Parental Discipline Strategies

In this chapter, relations between parental moral reasoning, child rearing, and children's moral reasoning are examined. First, the nature of moral reasoning and the stages of moral reasoning are described. Then a review is presented of the literature on factors affecting the development of moral reasoning in children. In this review, special attention is devoted to parental child-rearing behavior and discipline strategies. In a third introductory section, a rationale is presented for the assumed relations between the parents' level of moral reasoning, parental child rearing, and the development of moral reasoning in children.

The development and stimulation of a sense of moral values and norms can be considered a major task for primary and secondary socializing agents such as parents and teachers. In the literature, various theoretical explanations are offered for children's moral development. These explanations differ with regard to the aspects of moral development, and the emphasis on the processes underlying moral development (Shaffer & Brody, 1981; Gerris, 1988; Janssen, 1990). From a cognitive-structural point of view, children's judging and reasoning about moral standards for good or bad social behavior is emphasized. This study departs from this cognitive-structural perspective.

In this study, the development and stimulation of moral reasoning is investigated within the family context of parent-child interactions. However, it must be noted that according to Kohlberg (1969) "family participation is not unique or critically necessary for moral development, and the dimensions on which it stimulates moral development are primarily general dimensions by which other primary groups stimulate moral development" (pp. 399).

Four research questions are central to our study. First, which parental child-rearing behavior component is related to the development of the child's moral reasoning? Second, is this behavior component affected by the parents' level of moral reasoning? Third, is there empirical evidence of the hypothesis that parental child-rearing methods play a mediating role between the parents' and the child's level of moral reasoning? And finally, does the child rearing of both the father and the mother predict the child's moral development? By investigating these four questions, we expect to help answer the question of whether family participation should be considered as a unique or as a more general stimulating primary environment.

Moral values and standards can be viewed from various angles. In the first place, one can examine whether one's own moral reasoning represents specific moral values and standards. Such notions are called moral judgments, and judgment is passed on the virtuousness of specific actions. For example "stealing is wrong" or "you should help your fellow man". The second category of moral concepts comprises the arguments used to justify a particular moral judgment. The moral judgment "it is wrong to steal" can be approved of or disapproved of for different reasons: disapproval because it is to someone else's disadvantage, because the law forbids stealing, because people cannot trust each other anymore, or because one should not enrich oneself at the expense of a fellow man. But stealing can also be approved of because other people steal as well, because one will not be severely punished anyway, or because a thief also has to support a family. This category of moral cognitions is called "moral reasons". Because moral reasons are at the basis of moral judgments, these moral arguments also have a normative character.

According to Kohlberg (e.g. 1969, 1976, 1984), a taxonomy can be discovered in our reasoning about moral issues. Kohlberg argues that the taxonomy follows from the mental operations one executes to give meaning to the world. The mental operations relevant in this respect are connected with the nature of moral issues. Moral issues exist when a person's conduct is not in line with the claims, rights, obligations, values, standards, etc. of another person. In other words: if and when there is a social conflict situation.

A social conflict can only be perceived if one is capable of social perspective taking; the ability to associate attitudes of oneself and the other person (Selman, 1980; Gurucharri & Selman, 1982; Selman, Schorin, Stone & Phelps, 1983). There is ample evidence that the ability to take the other's perspective can adopt increasingly complex forms (Selman & Byrne, 1974; Selman, 1980; Gerris, 1981). The social perspective-taking skill is seen by Kohlberg (1976) and Selman (1976) as a necessary condition for moral reasoning. In addition, both Kohlberg (1976) and Selman (1976) explicate that reasoning about social reality is not the same as reasoning about moral reality. In Selman's words: "Moral judgment considers how people *should* think and act with regard to each other, while social role taking considers how and why people do *in fact* think about and act toward each other" (Selman, 1976, p. 307). For the practice of moral thinking in real-life situations, this distinction means that if people are capable of complex social perspective taking, this does not necessarily imply that they actually use this ability in moral thinking (see Selman, 1976). To distinguish the skill of social perspective taking in everyday social situations from the perspective taking ability in morally relevant situations, Kohlberg uses the term "sociomoral perspective taking": "...the (...) point of view from which the individual formulates moral judgments" (Colby, Kohlberg, Gibbs & Lieberman, 1983, p. 6). Sociomoral perspective taking moulds the moral reasoning at the basis of a particular moral judgment.

Kohlberg (1969, 1976, 1984) distinguished six sociomoral stages. Each stage is characterized by one form of sociomoral perspective taking, by which one can involve oneself or some other person in moral reasoning. The six sociomoral perspectives, each characterizing a stage of moral reasoning, can be placed in a developmental order. Each successive stage shows an increased moral-cognitive competence. The six stages will be dealt with very briefly. Extensive descriptions are presented by Kohlberg (1969, 1971, 1976, 1984).

The first stage reflects an egocentric point of view, which does not involve any differentiation between various ways of reasoning. Everybody is assumed to have the same perspective. And this perspective is determined by evident, superficial features of the situation or the person. Standards are viewed as having been stipulated externally by people who have the authority to do so. Hence this stage is called the stage of *heteronomous morality*. Examples of moral reasoning at this stage are: "One must not steal because stealing will lead to imprisonment"; "God always tells you to save someone else's life."

The second stage illustrates *individual and instrumental morality*. Each individual is assumed to have his own interests and behavior is assumed to be directed towards pursuing or defending these interests. Values and standards are derived from the expectation one has with regard to the satisfaction of his needs or the protection of his interests. For instance: "One is allowed to steal if one needs something"; "One does not have to save a person's life if one does not want to."

The third stage is characterized by *interpersonal normative morality*. It is the perspective of a person who is aware of his own interests, feelings, desires, needs as well as those of another person. At this stage, the subject is able to coordinate several perspectives. Examples of stage-3 reasoning are: "One must not steal, because by stealing one aggrieves somebody"; "One is supposed to save a person's life because everybody is expected to save lives."

In the fourth stage, the perspective does not refer to relations between persons, but to the relationship between persons and social institutions, such as society, the law, or religion. Norms regulate the cooperation and contribution of each individual. Kohlberg speaks of *the morality of the social system*. For example: "One must not steal, because society expects citizens not to"; "One should save someone's life because people are responsible for each other."

The fifth stage is characterized by the perspective of a person who is aware of the universal values and rights everyone would choose as appropriate foundations for a society. One has the idea there should be a consensus as to the nature of these values and standards. It is considered essential for any society that there be a certain extent of consensus on values, rights, obligations, and standards. This consensus is a basis for institutionalization in laws, cultural values and norms, and religious convictions. Kohlberg speaks of *morality of human rights and social welfare*. Examples of this perspective are: "If we want to coexist, we should not steal"; "Respect for each other's life constitutes the basis of our society."

The sixth stage, the stage of the *morality of universal ethical principles*, pertains to the perspective of a person who is aware of self-selected, abstract ethical principles. The solution of moral dilemmas is based on impartial, universal ethical principles, such as equality, reasonableness and reciprocity. For example: "All human beings are equal, and one should not draw any distinction when saving another person's life."

According to Kohlberg (1976), interaction with the social environment plays an important role in the development of moral reasoning. In interaction with others, one learns to take a more or less complex sociomoral perspective. According to Kohlberg (1976), three general factors may contribute to the development of moral reasoning: role-taking opportunities, moral atmosphere and cognitive-moral conflicts.

First, the development of moral reasoning is advanced when a person is frequently involved in situations that enable him or her to take social perspectives: situations in which one is confronted with the ideas, feelings, opinions, desires, needs, rights, duties, values and standards of other people. Kohlberg (1976) speaks of "role-taking opportunities". The skill of more complex social perspective taking is regarded as a necessary condition for more complex forms of sociomoral perspective taking.

Second, each social environment is characterized by the way fundamental rights and duties are distributed and decisions are taken (Kohlberg, Kaufman, Scharf & Hickey, 1975). In some environments, decisions are taken with reference to rules, traditions, the law or authority figures (stage-1 reasoning). In other environments, decisions are based on considerations as to what the system requires (stage 4 and higher). Kohlberg calls the stage of moral reasoning in a particular social environment the moral atmosphere of this environment. The stage of moral reasoning that is represented by a moral atmosphere stimulates people to reflect about moral values and norms.

A third factor that contributes to the development of moral reasoning is the occurrence of a cognitive-moral conflict: the confrontation of one's own moral reasoning with the reasoning of others. In a number of experimental studies, subjects were confronted with the moral reasoning of people who reasoned at a higher or lower stage. Children who were confronted with a stage of moral reasoning that was higher than their own exhibited a higher stage in the development of moral reasoning than children who were either confronted with moral reasoning of the same stage (Arbuthnot, 1975; Berkowitz, Gibbs & Broughton, 1980; Walker, 1982, 1983), or with moral reasoning of a lower stage (Arbuthnot, 1975; Norcini & Snyder, 1983), or with control groups that were not exposed to other people's moral reasoning (Arbuthnot, 1975; Walker, 1982).

From the theory and research summarized thus far, the hypothesis can be formulated that parents may stimulate the development of their children's moral reasoning by offering them the possibility of complex social perspective taking, by presenting a moral atmosphere representing a higher stage of moral reasoning, and by providing them with information that may lead to a moral-cognitive conflict, particularly by confronting their children with moral reasoning of a higher stage.

Within the parent-child interaction, various situations occur in which the three general factors mentioned above are found. For example, a discussion about values and standards, or an involvement of the child in decisions. Another apparently very important situation in which parents may influence their children's moral thinking occurs when a child offends a value or norm, and the parents discipline the child for doing so. Parental child-discipline encounters of this kind occur very frequently (Clifford, 1959; Simons & Schoggen, 1963; Minton, Kagan & Levine, 1971; Hoffman, 1983; Schaffer, 1984). Such encounters appear to occur in daily family life as a result of a wide range of norm transgressions (Clifford, 1959; Brown, Cunningham & Birkimer, 1983; Hawley, Shear, Stark & Goodman, 1984; Ellis-Schwabe & Thornburg, 1985; Hakim-Larson, Livingstone & Tron, 1985; Vermulst, Gerris, Franken & Janssens, 1986; Hill & Holmbeck, 1987; Papini, 1987; Pettit & Bayles, 1987). There is ample evidence that norm transgressions are part of daily parent-child interaction during a long period, ranging from the age of two until deep in middle childhood and pre-adolescence. Therefore, parental disciplining reactions may be considered very relevant to the development of child's moral thinking. Especially if it pertains to the transgression of a moral value or standard, as opposed to transgressions of domestic rules (Smetana, 1989). Transgressions of moral values and standards are considered relevant because disciplining reactions show what moral values and norms parents consider important.

In view of the frequent occurrence and the relevance of disciplining reactions, in this study attention is solely devoted to how parents may influence their children's development of moral reasoning by way of their disciplining behavior.

What reactions do parents have after the occurrence of a transgression? A number of disciplinary techniques can be distinguished (Clifford, 1959; Hoffman, 1970; Minton et al., 1971; Magmer & Ipfling, 1973; Conroy, Hess, Azuma & Kashiwagi, 1980; Grusec & Kucszynski, 1984; Mladek, 1982; Zahn-Waxler & Chapman, 1982; Kuczynski, 1984; Oldenshaw, Walters & Hall, 1986; Trickett & Kuczynski, 1986; Kuczynski, Kochanska, Radke-Yarrow & Girnius-Brown, 1987; Trickett & Susman, 1988). Analysis of the research literature resulted in the following categories of disciplinary techniques and strategies:
– *Ignoring the transgression.*
– *Verbal, disapproving reaction.* For example, overt disapproval of behavior ("Hitting is not allowed"), ridiculing the child, scolding, appealing to the child's self-esteem ("So you really think you're a

big guy?"), or explicitly expressing disappointment about the child's behavior .

- *Commanding*. Parents may order the child to immediately adhere to a norm by forbidding or compelling behavior. Grusec and Kuczynski (1980), Mladek (1982) and Kuczynski et al. (1987) distinguish between friendly requests and commands. According to Minton et al. (1971), commands can be given indirectly (e.g. by calling the child's name, or by means of "Hey!"), by a simple prohibition ("Stop that!"; "Stop!"), or by indicating explicitly what is required ("Clean up the table"). Kuczynski et al. (1987) add nonverbal command to this list, such as looking at the child in a compelling manner.
- *Punishment*. A number of studies distinguish between physical and non-physical punishment (Clifford, 1959; Minton et al., 1971; Magmer & Ipfling, 1973; Zahn-Waxler & Chapman, 1982; Oldenshaw et al., 1986; Trickett & Kuczynski, 1986; Trickett & Susman, 1988). Physical punishment refers to parental behavior that causes pain or fear, for example by hitting or kicking. Non-physical punishment means the parent refuses something the child likes (e.g. privileges, food, toys, money, affection, the liberty to go where one likes, etc.) or confronts the child with something he or she evaluates negatively (e.g. school punishment, scaring, extra domestic tasks, being put to bed early). Clifford's (1959) "restitution" category (compensating for damage) can also be regarded as a form of punishment. At any rate, a number of studies distinguish between the actual assignment of punishment and the threat of punishment .
- *Giving information*. The following specific forms are mentioned: making it clear why the child must obey, referring to one's authority or to non-personal characteristics of the situation (e.g., "If you don't clean up now, the table cannot be set"), informing the child about the material, emotional, or social consequences of the transgression for someone else, informing the child about important values and norms, explaining what is required in similar situations, pointing out the characteristics of the situation ("don't do that; we have guests") or referring to a previous or similar experience.
- *Diverting the child*. The parent focusses the child's attention on other matters.
- *Positive reaction to transgression*. For example, flattering, praising, approving, soothing, showing signs of affection, or laughing.
- *Questioning the child's motives*. The parent asks the child about the

reasons for his or her behavior, for example "Why did you do that?"
- *Negative physical intervention*. The parent clasps the child tightly to add force to demands.

What is the potential effect of these disciplinary strategies on the development of a child's moral reasoning? In order to infer empirical hypotheses about this relationship, Kohlberg's three above-mentioned general factors are used as criteria.

First of all, a stimulating influence can be expected when a particular discipline technique gives the child an opportunity for social perspective taking. This is the case when another person's position or role is explained in a norm-transgressing situation. For instance, by pointing out that other people experience a situation differently, or by referring to the thoughts, feelings, intentions, etc. of other persons.

Second, one can assume that parental discipline techniques are strongly related to the moral atmosphere within the family. When a parent threatens to hit a child or send a child to bed, the child is confronted with an egocentric, authoritarian perspective-taking characteristic of stage-1 reasoning. When a parent points out the consequences of the transgression for the victim, and demands that the child take into account the victim's interest, the transgressor is confronted with the demand for the coordination of individual perspectives, which is characteristic of the third stage of moral reasoning.

Third, one can assume that particular parental discipline strategies cause a moral-cognitive conflict within the child. This may be the case when the parental information and reasoning refer to a higher stage of moral reasoning than the child's stage of reasoning.

Based on these three criteria, one can analyze which of the nine distinguished discipline reactions exert a stimulating influence on the development of a child's moral reasoning. *Ignoring the child's transgression, Diverting the child or Reacting positively to a transgression* do not seem to offer an opportunity for perspective taking, do not say anything about the way rights and duties are regulated, and do not stimulate a cognitive conflict because these disciplinary techniques do not confront the child with moral ideas of a higher stage of moral reasoning. *Verbally disapproving of the child, ordering the child to do something or to abstain from doing something, administering punishment and interfering physically* are types of disciplining reactions that only indicate to the child that the parent has a different opinion about the child's behavior, but without contributing to the process of learning to reflect on what the victim thinks or how he or she feels about the transgression. An exception has to be made for disciplinary reactions that confront the child with the material or emotional loss that a victim has suffered due to the transgression, for instance when the parent wants the child to apologize, or to pay for the damage or repair it. Hoffman (1984) notes that disapproving, demanding, or punishing reactions confront a child with the consequences of the transgression for himself or herself. Therefore, these reactions hardly offer an opportunity for of social perspective taking. They convey the message that particular actions by the child have a moral dimension, since an authority formulates rules about these actions or administers punishment for them. These four disciplinary techniques (*Verbally disapproving of the child, ordering the child to do something or to abstain from doing something, administering punishment and interfering physically*) are summarized by means of the category "power assertion". Power-assertive reactions represent stage-1 reasoning. Perhaps an exception should be made for reactions that demand correction from the child. They convey the message that certain behavior is morally reprehensible because it damages other persons, and that this should be taken into consideration (stage-3 reasoning). But verbally disapproving of the child's behavior, ordering the child to do something or to abstain from doing something, administering punishment, and physically interfering are reactions that, according to the theory, do not stimulate the child's development of moral reasoning.

On the other hand, reactions anticipating that the child will correct his or her behavior seem to have a potentially stimulating value. Reactions that provide the child with information may also stimulate his or her development of moral reasoning. The child is offered an opportunity for perspective taking when the parent indicates what the consequences of the transgression are for the victim, the parent, or the (non-disciplinary) consequences for himself (e.g. "If you act like that, he won't trust you anymore"); when one refers to similar or previous experiences of the child ("You wouldn't want him to break one of your things either, would you?"), and when a positive norm is formulated that indicates how to behave in a socially and morally acceptable manner ("You must try to share and share alike so that each of you gets the same"). In giving information of this kind, the parent creates a moral atmosphere in which the other person's perspective is involved (stage-3 reasoning or higher). The parent does so by referring to the perspective of others or to matters that play an important role within a relation (stage-3 reasoning or higher), which might potentially lead to a moral-cognitive conflict on the child's part. *Questioning* promotes the cognitive processing of matters that played a role in a transgression situation (Berkowitz & Gibbs, 1983; Peterson & Skevington, 1987) and may therefore allow a moral-cognitive conflict to occur. Hence questioning may also be regarded as a stimulus for the child's development of moral reasoning. In view of the potential power of questioning and providing the child with information to stimulate his development of moral reasoning, these techniques will be labelled "induction".

As a result of the above-mentioned rationale, the developmental stage of the child's moral reasoning can be expected to be positively related to parental use of induction. Hoffman (1984) points out that parents usually use more than one disciplinary technique in a situation. A parent may point out the emotional condition of the victim and, in addition, punish the child severely. According to Hoffman (1983, 1984), the resistance, anger or fear that power assertion evokes may interfere with an effective processing of the information conveyed in the inductive reaction. Induction may only be effective if it takes place within a context of restricted power assertion (cf. Lepper, 1983). Based on these ideas, we hypothesize that the developmental stage of a child's moral reasoning depends on the extent to which his parents use relatively many inductive reactions as reactions to transgressions of norms, and abstain from strongly power-assertive disciplinary techniques.

Why are some parents more power-assertive, whereas others use inductive disciplinary techniques more frequently? In this study, we try to explain differences in parental disciplining strategies on the basis of differences in parental moral reasoning. A transgression requires a parental normative judgment about a child's behavior. So far, we have argued that parental normative judgments may be based on the stage of moral reasoning. The parent's stage of moral reasoning therefore seems to be an important determinant of his or her discipline behavior. Parents who are capable of formulating moral arguments representing a higher stage of moral reasoning will probably also be able to express these arguments in the information they give their child. A parent who takes the view that one should be considerate of others (stage-3 reasoning) will be more apt to refer to the victim of the child's transgression. Parents who reason about moral issues at a higher stage, may react to a child's transgression in such a way that the child's development of moral reasoning is stimulated. This hypothesis seems to be confirmed by the research results of Olejnik

(1980) and Parikh (1980). In a study involving 50 students (men and women), Olejnik noted a positive relation between the stage of moral reasoning and the extent to which the students said they preferred inductive disciplining-reactions, as well as a negative relation between their stage of moral reasoning and the preference for the use of power-assertive reactions. With a group of 39 mothers, Parikh noted a positive relation between the mothers' stage of moral reasoning and their use of inductive reactions to transgressions by their children. This relation also exists when the extent of induction has been based on data supplied by their children. Based on these results, we hypothesize that parents who reason about moral issues at higher stages use more inductive and less power-assertive disciplinary techniques than parents who reason at lower stages.

Method

Subjects
The sample consisted of 124 families in the East and South of the Netherlands. In each family, the father, mother and one child, aged nine to thirteen, participated in the study. The sample consisted of approximately equal numbers of skilled workers, lower, intermediate, and higher employees (Van Westerlaak, Kropman & Collaris, 1975).

Instruments
Stage of moral reasoning of parent and child. The stage of moral reasoning of the children and parents was assessed with a translated and adapted version of Gibbs and Widaman's "Sociomoral Reflection Measure" (SRM) (1982). The SRM consists of two parallel versions, which are psychometrically equivalent (Gibbs & Widaman, 1982). We used the most frequently applied A-version, which contains the famous Heinz dilemma. In each story, a moral dilemma gives rise to a number of questions. Each question is meant to elicit the respondent's most competent stage of moral reasoning. The questions refer to eight moral value areas: marriage or friendship, the value of life, law; justice, conscience, solidarity between child and educator, contract, and the power of disposal of possessions.

From a pilot study, it was clear that a large number of children had problems in understanding the phrasing of the SRM questions. Therefore, a linguistically adapted and simplified child-version was used for this study. A second adaptation refers to the use of cartoons.

In order to make the story more concrete and to give the respondents a mnemonic aid when answering the questions, a number of drawings were shown while they read each story. A final adaptation pertained to the contents of the two stories. Because of the typically American nature of the second story (a father who reconsiders his promise to go camping with his son) has been changed into a situation more recognizable for Dutch children (a parent who reconsiders a promise to let the child go to the fair). Furthermore, a female leading figure was involved in the dilemma of each story so as not to give the impression that moral dilemmas only take place among men. Parents were separately interviewed at home and children were interviewed at school. All the interviews were audiotaped and transcribed verbatim.

Each statement was tested for one or more moral arguments. When a statement did not seem to contain any, it was considered unscorable. When a moral reason was scorable, the stage of moral reasoning represented by that argument was assessed (inter-rater reliability varied between 0.76 and 0.93, dependent on moral value area). For each moral value area, the highest score was assessed. Then a mean was computed based on these highest scores.

Parental disciplining reactions. To assess parental use of power assertion and induction, we also interviewed both parents. They were asked to imagine ten concrete discipline situations in which their child transgressed a norm and we asked them what they would do or say. All the answers were audiotaped and transcribed. The parents usually gave more than one reaction to each situation. The reactions of each parent to each situation were coded with the coding system represented in Table 1 (inter-rater reliability = 0.77). The coding system listed 22 disciplinary techniques based on the above-mentioned nine categories of child discipline. For each situation, we counted the reactions that were power-assertive and those that were inductive. Power-assertive reactions included physical punishment or the threat of it, punishment or the threat of it, isolation, ignoring actively, physical intervention, and parental demands to do something or abstain from doing something immediately. Inductive reactions included: demanding that the transgressor apologizes, sincerely questioning the transgressor, pointing out the material, financial, emotional or social consequences of the transgression for the victim or the parent, pointing out the material, financial, emotional or social consequences of the transgression for the transgressor himself, having the transgressor put himself in the position of another person, refering to reciprocity in the relationship, and giving other explanations of the situation.

Table 1   List of disciplinary reactions

A	**Ignoring the transgression.**
A1	The parent decides not to discipline.

B	**Verbal, disapproving reactions.**
B1	Repudiating the transgressor's behavior.
B2	Rejecting the transgressor.
B3	The parent emphasizes that the child is responsible for the transgression.

C	**Commanding.**
C1	Demand that the transgressor has to do something or hast to abstain from doing something immediately.
C2	Demand that the transgressor apologizes for the transgression.
C3	Demand that the transgressor pays for the damage materially or financially or cleans up the damage.
C4	Demand that the transgressor carries out an order again.

D	**Punishment.**
D1	Physical punishment or threat of it.
D2	Punishment or threat of it.
D3	Isolation or sending transgressor to his/her room or threat to do so.
D4	Ignoring the transgressor in an active manner.

E	**Giving information.**
E1	Stressing the material, financial, emotional or social consequences of the transgression for the victim or the parent.
E2	Stressing the material, financial, emotional or social consequences for the transgressor.
E3	The parent has the transgressor put himself/herself in another person's position.
E4	The parent refers to reciprocity in the relationship.
E5	Other explanations.
E6	Confronting the transgressor with a positively formulated social norm.
E7	Confronting the transgressor with a positively formulated non-social norm.

F	Diverting the transgressor.
G	Positive reaction to transgression.
H	Questioning the motives of the transgressor.
I	Physical intervention by the parent.

Following Hoffman's suggestion, we assumed that a moderate form of power-assertion should be embedded in a mainly inductive strategy, and this would have a stimulating effect on the development of the child's moral reasoning. For this purpose, a so called discipline score was computed for each situation: the difference between the number of inductive techniques used in a situation and the number of power-assertive reactions used in the same situation. The tendency of parents to use induction or power-assertion in different transgression situations can be expressed in a mean score based on the ten situation scores. Previous research showed that disciplining is situationally determined (Conroy, Hess, Azuma, & Kashiwagi, 1980; Grusec & Kuczynski, 1980; Mladek, 1982; Grusec, Dix & Mills, 1982; Wolfe, Katell & Drabman, 1982; Zahn-Waxler & Chapman, 1982; Smetana, 1984; Reid & Valsinger, 1986; Siebenheller, 1990). We wanted to see whether that also applied to our combined discipline score. Therefore, a 10 (situations) * 2 (parents) ANOVA, with situation and parent as within-subjects factors, was carried out. Important situational effects were noted for the discipline score ($F(9,97) = 7.40$, $p < 0.01$). Discipline is therefore considered as situationally determined. This means the scores per situation were not comparable because of the different probability of induction and power-assertion being applied in a particular situation. Therefore the scores were transformed to z-scores per situation. Moreover, the analysis showed a significant difference between fathers and mothers ($F(1,105) = 115.31$, $p < 0.01$). Fathers and mothers thus differed in the extent to which they applied inductive and power-assertive discipline techniques. Therefore, the z-transformation per situation had to take place separately for fathers and mothers. From the ten parental z-scores, a mean score was computed. The higher that score, the more a parent uses induction and the less he or she uses overt power assertion.

Results

In Table 2, Pearson correlations between the paternal and the maternal stage of moral reasoning, the paternal and the maternal discipline, and the child's stage of moral reasoning are presented. Both the paternal and the maternal stage of moral reasoning were positively related to the discipline strategy; The higher the stage at which parents reasoned about moral issues, the more they used inductive disciplinary techniques and the less they relied on power assertion.

Child discipline was also positively related to the child's stage of moral reasoning. Children whose parents favored inductive discipline techniques, reasoned at higher stages than children whose parents preferred power assertive discipline.

Table 2   Correlations Between Maternal and Paternal Moral Reasoning, Maternal and Paternal Discipline, and the Child's Stage of Moral Reasoning

	MMR	PMR	MD	PD
Maternal moral reasoning (MMR)	–			
Paternal moral reasoning (PMR)	0.31*	–		
Maternal discipline (MD)	0.33*	0.19*	–	
Paternal discipline (PD)	-0.01	0.28*	0.25*	–
Child's moral reasoning	0.26*	0.17*	0.32*	0.28*

* $p < 0.05$

To analyze whether child discipline mediated between the parental stage of moral reasoning and the child's stage of moral reasoning, data were analyzed with LISREL-analysis. We tested the model presented in Figure 1. The model did not fit the data (Chi-square = 13.90, d.f. = 5, p = 0.016). Modification indices indicated that the model could be improved by introducing a relation between paternal and maternal discipline. To test a second model, the LISREL-program was used to estimate the unexplained covariance between parental and maternal discipline. Modification indices also indicated that there was a direct effect of the maternal stage of moral reasoning on the child's stage of moral reasoning. This direct effect was also estimated by way of a second model (see Figure 2). The overall-fit of this model was satisfactory (Chi-square = 2.12, d.f. = 3, p = 0.548). In Figure 2, the strength of the relations between the variables in the model is represented by the

standardized regression coefficients along the arrows. All the estimated regression coefficients were statistically significant (p < 0.01).
Figure 2 shows that parental discipline depends on the parental stage
of moral reasoning. Parents who reasoned about moral issues at a
higher stage were more inductive and less power assertive than
parents who reasoned at lower stages. Use of induction had a positive
effect on the child's level of moral reasoning. From these results, we
concluded that parental discipline mediates between the parent's and
the child's stage of moral reasoning. But the influence of maternal
moral reasoning on the child's level of moral reasoning was not only
mediated by maternal discipline. There was also a direct effect of
moral reasoning about moral issues on the child's stage of reasoning
about these issues.

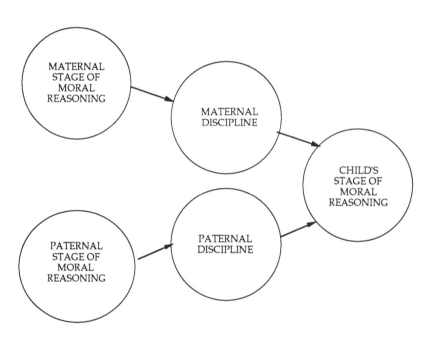

Figure 1   Model to explain child's stage of moral reasoning

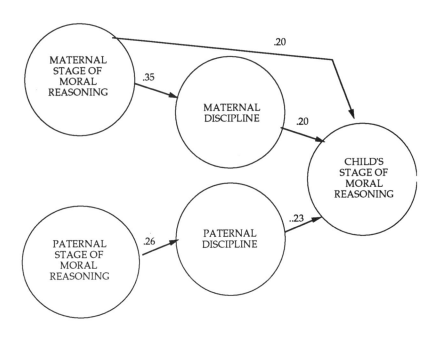

Figure 2   Child's stage of moral reasoning explained from parental discipline

Discussion

Four research questions were central to this study. First, which parental child-rearing behavior component is related to the development of a child's moral reasoning? Second, is this behavior component affected by the parents' level of moral reasoning? Third, is there any empirical evidence to back the hypothesis that parental child-rearing methods play a mediating role between parents' and children's levels of moral reasoning? And finally, does the child rearing of both the father and the mother predict the child's moral development?

The first research question pertained to the relation between child-rearing behavior and the development of a child's moral reasoning. On the basis of a theoretical analysis, it was assumed that a positive influence may be attached to inductive discipline in a slightly power assertive context. Although a causal relation cannot be demonstrated within the chosen research design, the assumed relation has indeed

been noted.This finding supports the assumption that inductive discipline techniques constitute a potential source of stimulation for the
development of a child's sociomoral perspective taking and of the
stage of his moral reasoning.

The positive relations between the parental discipline score and the
stage of a child's moral reasoning implies that a cognitive-structural
approach to the development of moral reasoning is complementary to
a socialization-theoretical point of view (cf. Peterson, Hey & Peterson,
1979; Gibbs & Schnell, 1985).This meant that researchers and theorists
should be open to the effects of parental behavior on the development
of the structural characteristics of a child's thinking. Kohlberg (1976)
saw the influence of the family primarily in the area of family
discussions about values and norms "rather than by specific experiences with parents or experiences of discipline, punishment, and
reward" (1976, p. 48). This study tends to imply that the cognitive-
structural quality of specific discipline-experiences most certainly
plays a role in the development of a child's moral reasoning. Thus,
discipline situations are a special or unique category of situations
within parent-child interaction that may have a substantial influence
on a child's development of moral reasoning. In this sense, the results
do not fit Kohlberg's position. On the other hand, the dimensions and
mechanisms that stimulate moral reasoning within a disciplinary
context are general rather than unique, and in this sense our results
support Kohlberg's position.
The finding that inductive discipline plays a role in the development
of a child's moral reasoning requires some further elaboration in view
of the theoretical considerations and the psychological meaning of the
score used. This study shows that induction only appears to contribute to the development of a child's moral reasoning if the parent
applies power assertion to a limited extent. In a related study conducted by Janssen (1990), it was shown that if stronger use of power is
made, a higher stage of moral reasoning is no longer explained by the
parent's use of induction. Apparently, the context in which induction
occurs emanates an important moderating influence on the development of a child's moral reasoning. This finding is in accordance with
the ideas of Hoffman (1984) and Radke-Yarrow, Zahn-Waxler and
Chapman (1983), that attention should be devoted to the interactive
effect of different dimensions of child rearing on a child's development. According to Hoffman (1984), with regard to the use of power-
assertion and induction by the parent, the underlying process is that
power assertion interferes with a sufficiently cognitive processing of

the inductive message. There are some indications of the course of this process. Research has shown that an adult's anger evokes strong, negative reactions in the child. This is shown by the child's behavior, such as anger or recalcitrance, but also by the measurement of physiological reactions. This is not only the case when the anger is directed against some person other than the child (Cummings, Zahn-Waxler & Radke-Yarrow, 1984; Cummings, 1987; Cummings, Pellegrini, Notarius & Cummings, 1989; El-Sheikh, Cummings & Goetsch, 1989), but even more so when the child is the object of the parental anger. Research by Crockenberg (1985) shows that parental anger, especially directed against the child, brings about an increased anger or provoking behavior on the part of the child, and a virtual lack of any concern whatsoever for anyone else's fate. These findings support Hoffman's claim that an angry and punishing parent evokes reactions in the child that inhibit him from being open to the cognitive processing of a possibly inductive message from the parent.

The second question was whether parental discipline depends on the extent to which the parent has reached a higher stage of moral reasoning. The results show that this question can also be answered affirmatively. The results do not contradict the assumption that the moral-cognitive structure of the parent is largely responsible for the parental disciplinary reaction. For it is the frequent use of induction as a disciplinary technique that demands from the parent that he discerns the complexity of social perspectives and integrate them into a situation of social conflict. Besides, Powers (1988) indicates that parents who are capable of more complex moral reasoning also tend to take the complexity of moral dilemmas into consideration, and explain contradictions. Moreover, these parents seem to be better advocates of their own moral arguments.

The third question was whether parental child-rearing methods play a mediating role between the parents' and the child's level of moral reasoning. As was expected, the relation that was found elsewhere (Buck, Walsh & Rothman, 1981; Haan, Langer & Kohlberg, 1976; Holstein, 1972; Parikh, 1980; Speicher, 1985a; Walker, 1989) between the parental and the child's stage of moral reasoning appeared to be mediated by the quality of the parental disciplinary reaction. Furthermore, the LISREL-analysis shows that there is also a direct relation between the mother's and the child's stage of moral reasoning. This means that the mother also influences the child's stage of moral reasoning in one or more alternative ways other than by discipline behavior. A number of possibilities can be mentioned.

A first possibility is that the mother expresses her stage of moral reasoning by means of moral discussions with the child that do not fall within the context of norm-transgressions or discipline encounters (Speicher, 1985b). A second possibility is that the mother's stage of moral reasoning is strongly related to the moral atmosphere within the family (Holstein, 1972). A third possibility is that the child becomes acqainted with the mother's more complex moral reasoning because the child observes interactions between the mother and other people. It is known that children focus their attention on the disciplinary interaction between the parent and a norm-transgressing brother or sister at a very early age, especially in the case of norm-transgressions (Dunn & Munn, 1985).

Regarding the fourth and final question, both the paternal and the maternal discipline process appear to be positively related with the stage of moral reasoning of the child. Besides, for both groups of parents the disciplinary process appears to be partially explained by their stage of moral reasoning. Within the scope of the present research, the only difference between fathers and mothers appears to exist in the ways the stages of parental and children's moral reasoning are connected. For fathers, this relation is mediated by their disciplinary behavior. The stage of moral reasoning is also connected with the child's stage of moral reasoning through mechanisms other than child-discipline. This finding seems to confirm the important socializing role that may be attributed to mothers.

We might wonder whether or not efforts on the child rearers' part to stimulate a child's development of moral reasoning should be regarded as desirable. Kohlberg (1971) not only assigns a developmental-psychological dimension to his developmental model, but a normative one as well; attaining a higher stage of moral reasoning not only means a better use of cognitive abilities, it also means an ethical improvement. According to Kohlberg, this is a consequence of the fact that before one can reach a successive stage, one has to be able to distinguish between the viewpoints of various people involved in a moral dilemma, and also that one has to be able to integrate the viewpoints in a better way.

Kohlberg's argument that, each successive stage is thus "more moral" can be refuted on logical grounds: "[The moral principle of justice (...) undoubtedly assumes the necessary role-taking ability from the persons involved, but an increasing ability to be considerate of other people's viewpoints and interests does of course by no means guarantee that that will happen in a just manner.]" (Van Haaften, 1984).

What arguments can be put forward to demonstrate that the development of moral reasoning is desirable? In other words, why is a higher moral stage desired from a moral point of view? The answer that follows is based on the frequent observation that moral reasoning by adolescents is connected negatively with what is generally considered to be morally reprehensible behavior. Examples of this are deceit (Kohlberg & Candee, 1984), aggressiveness (Bear & Richards, 1989) and delinquent behavior (for a review of relevant studies before 1980, see: Jurkovic, 1980 and Blasi, 1980; Gavaghan, Arnold & Gibbs, 1983; Schnell & Gibbs, 1987; Trevethan & Walker, 1989). Arbuthnot and Gordon (1986) have empirically shown that vandalism and delinquent behavior can be drastically decreased by stimulating the development of young people's moral reasoning. Apart from being connected with undesirable behavior, the stage of moral reasoning appears to be positively correlated with desirable behavior, such as altruistic behavior (Blasi, 1980).

The assumption (Gibbs, Arnold, Morgan, Schwatrz, Gavaghan & Tappan, 1984) is that higher stages provide a "cognitive buffer" against anti-social influences and temptations. In other words, a higher stage of moral reasoning, based on more complex sociomoral perspective-taking does not fit the idea of the serious, psycho-social (Smale, 1980), financial, material, and/or social consequences of crimes, and it certainly does not fit the generally accepted morally and legally institutionalized norm which says that one should not damage other persons or inflict injuries on them. Research results provide support for the assumption by Gibbs et al.: the expectation that one damages other persons (Perry, Perry & Rasmussen, 1986) and the importance one attaches to sparing other persons suffering (Slaby & Guerra, 1988; Boldizar, Perry & Perry, 1989) indeed appear to be important antecedents of non-aggressive behavior in young people. Because of this correlation between moral behavior and moral reasoning, there may be some arguments for the position that it is better for the child to attain as high a stage of moral reasoning as possible.

The research results show that a child's development of moral reasoning can be stimulated in different ways. First, by interfering with parental disciplinary actions. The parents should react in a more inductive way to norm transgressions, and should also act in a less power-assertive manner. It has been found that parental disciplinary reactions can be changed in the desired direction (Stanley, 1978, 1980; Lickona, 1980)

In the second place, by interfering with the factors that contribute to a more inductive and less power-assertive reaction. The stage of moral reasoning appears to provide a major contribution to this discipline strategy. The development of the stage of moral reasoning is promoted by means of discussion groups (Blatt & Kohlberg, 1975; Berkowitz & Gibbs, 1983) and role plays (Arbuthnot, 1975; Matefy & Acksen, 1976; Walker, 1982; 1983).

If parental disciplinary reactions are of importance to the development of children's moral reasoning, it may well be that particular groups of children run the risk of lagging behind in the development of moral reasoning. Examples are the children of parents who react in a relatively strong power-assertive manner, as may be the case with parents in a divorce conflict (Hetherington, 1981) or some single-parent families (Gerris, Vermulst, Franken & Janssens, 1986; Vermulst et al., 1986), child-abusing parents (Trickett & Kuczynski, 1986; Trickett & Susman, 1988) and parents of children who are difficult to handle (Mullhern & Passman, 1981; Patterson, 1981; 1982). Both parents and counseling agencies and schools should be aware of the consequences of a child-rearing strategy dominated by power assertion for the development of moral reasoning of these groups of children.

References

Arbuthnot, J. (1975). Modification of moral judgment through role playing. *Developmental Psychology, 11*, 319-324.

Arbuthnot, J. & Gordon, D.A. (1986). Behavioral and cognitive effects of a moral reasoning development intervention for high-risk behavior-disordered adolescents. *Journal of Consulting and Clinical Psychology, 54*, 208-216.

Bear, G.G. & Richards, H.C. (1989). Sociomoral reasoning and aggressive behaviors in the regular classroom: A replication. Paper presented at the Biennial Meeting of the Society for Research in Child Development. Kansas City, MO.

Berkowitz, M.W., Gibbs, J.C. & Broughton, J.M. (1980). The relation of moral judgment stage disparity to developmental effects of peer dialogues. *Merrill-Palmer Quarterly, 26*, 341-357.

Berkowitz, M.W. & Gibbs, J.C. (1983). Measuring the developmental features of moral discussion. *Merrill-Palmer Quarterly, 29*, 399-410.

Blasi, A. (1980). Bridging moral cognition and moral action: A critical review of the literature. *Psychological Bulletin, 88*, 1-45.

Blatt, M.M. & Kohlberg, L. (1975). The effects of classroom moral discussion upon children's level of moral judgment. *Journal of Moral Education, 4*, 129-161.

Boldizar, J.P., Perry, D.G. & Perry, L.C. (1989). Outcome values and aggression. *Child Development, 60(3)*, 571-579.

Brown, J.H., Cunningham, G. & Birkimer, J.C. (1983). A telephone home survey to identify parent-child problems and maintaining conditions. *Child and Family Behavior Therapy, 5*, 85-92.

Buck, L.Z., Walsh, W. & Rothman, G. (1981). Relationship between parental moral judgment and socialization. *Youth and Society, 13*, 91-116.

Clifford, E. (1959). Discipline in the home: A controlled observational study of parental practices. *Journal of Genetic Psychology, 95*, 45-82.

Colby, A., Kohlberg, L., Gibbs, J. & Lieberman, M. (1983). A longitudinal study of moral development. *Monographs of the Society for Research in Child Development, 48(1, Serial No. 200)*.

Conroy, M., Hess, R.D., Azuma, H. & Kashiwagi, K. (1980). Maternal strategies for regulating children's behavior. *Journal of Cross-cultural Psychology, 11*, 153-172.

Crockenberg, S. (1985). Toddlers' reactions to maternal anger. *Merrill-Palmer Quarterly, 31*, 361-373.

Cummings, E.M. (1987). Coping with background anger in early childhood. *Child Development, 58(4)*, 976-984.

Cummings, E.M., Zahn-Waxler, C. & Radke-Yarrow, M. (1984). Developmental changes in children's reactions to anger in the home. *Journal of Consulting and Clinical Psychology, 25(1)*, 63-74.

Cummings, J.S., Pellegrini, D.S. & Notarius, C.I. (1989). Children's response to angry adult behavior as a function of marital distress and history of interparent hostility. *Child Development, 60(5)*, 1035-1043.

Dunn, J. & Munn, P. (1985). Becoming a family member: Family conflict and the development of social understanding in the second year. *Child Development, 56*, 480-492.

Ellis-Schwabe, M. & Thornburg, H.D. (1985). Conflict areas between parents and their adolescents. *Journal of Psychology, 120(1)*, 59-68.

El-Sheikh, C.E.M. & Goetsch, V.L. (1989). Coping with adults' angry behavior: Behavioral, physiological, and verbal responses in preschoolers. *Developmental Psychology, 25(4)*, 490-498.

Gavaghan, M.P., Arnold, K.D. & Gibbs, J.C. (1983). Moral judgment in delinquents and nondelinquents: Recognition versus production measures. *Journal of Psychology, 114*, 267-274.

Gerris, J.R.M. (1981). *Onderwijs en sociale ontwikkeling: Een tijdreeksonderzoek naar de effecten van een onderwijsprogramma voor sociale cognitie.* Lisse: Swets & Zeitlinger.

Gerris, J.R.M. (1988). Bevordering van de socio-morele ontwikkeling. *Justitiële Verkenningen, 14(8)*, 60-69.

Gerris, J.R.M., Vermulst, A.A., Franken, W.M. & Janssens, J.M.A.M. (1986). Social class and parental situation perceptions as determinants of parental value orientations and behaviors. Paper presented at the second European Conference on Developmental Psychology, 10-13 September 1986, Rome, Italy.

Gibbs, J.C., Arnold, K.D., Morgan, R.L., Schwartz, E.S., Gavaghan, M.P. & Tappan, M.B. (1984). Construction and validation of a multiple-choice measure of moral reasoning. *Child Development, 55*, 527-536.

Gibbs, J.C. & Schnell, S.V. (1985). Moral development versus socialization: A critique. Paper presented at the Biennial Meeting of the Society for Research in Child Development. Toronto.

Gibbs, J.C. & Widaman, K.F. (1982). *Social intelligence: Measuring the development of sociomoral reflection.* Englewood Cliffs, NJ: Prentice-Hall.

Grusec, J.E., Dix, T. & Mills, R. (1982). The effects of type, severity, and victim of children's transgressions on maternal discipline. *Canadian Journal of Behavioral Science, 14*, 276-289.

Grusec, J.E. & Kuczynski, L. (1980). Direction of effect in socialization: A comparison of the parent vs. the child's behavior as determinants of disciplinary techniques. *Developmental Psychology, 16(1)*, 1-9.

Gurucharri, C., Phelps, E. & Selman, R. (1984). Development of interpersonal understanding: A longitudinal and comparative study of normal and disturbed youths. *Journal of Consulting and Clinical Psychology, 52*, 26-36.

Haaften, A.W.van (1984). De 'is-ought question'. *Pedagogische Studiën, 61*, 261-271.

Haan, N., Langer, J. & Kohlberg, L. (1976). Family patterns of moral reasoning. *Child Development, 47*, 1204-1206.

Hakim-Larson, J. & Livingston, J. (1985). Mothers and adolescent daughters: Personal issues of conflict and congruency. Paper presented at the Biennial Meeting of the Society for Research in Child Development. Toronto.

Hawley, L.E., Shear, C.L., Stark, A.M. & Goodman, P.R. (1984). Resident and parental perceptions of adolescent problems and family communications in a low socioeconomic population. *Journal of Family Practice, 19*, 652-655.

Hetherington, E.M. (1980). Children and divorce. In R.W. Henderson (Ed.), *Parent-child interaction. Theory, research, and prospects.* New York: Academic Press.

Hill, J.P. & Holmbeck, G.N. (1987). Disagreement about rules in families with seventh-grade girls and boys. *Journal of Youth and Adolescence, 16(3)*, 221-246.

Hoffman, M.L. (1970). Conscience, personality, and socialization techniques. *Human Development, 13*, 90-126.

Hoffman, M.L. (1983). Affective and cognitive processes in moral internalization. In E.T. Higgins, D.N. Ruble, & W.W. Hartup (Eds.), *Social cognition and social development. A sociocultural perspective.* Cambridge: Cambridge University Press.

Hoffman, M.L. (1984). Parent discipline, moral internalization, and development of prosocial motivation. In E. Staub, D. Bar-Tal, J. Karyloski, & J. Reykowski (Eds.), *Development and maintenance of prosocial behavior.* New York: Plenum Press.

Holstein, C.E. (1972). The relation of children's moral judgment level to that of their parents and to communication patterns in the family. In R. Smart, & M. Smart (Eds.), *Readings in child development and relationships.* (pp. 484-494). New York: MacMillan.

Janssen, A.W.H. (1990). *"Ik zal je mores leren!" Een onderzoek naar de relatie tussen opvoedergedrag en de morele ontwikkeling van het kind.* Dissertation, Catholic University of Nijmegen.

Jurkovic, G.J. (1980). The juvenile delinquent as a moral philosopher: A structural-developmental perspective. *Psychological Bulletin, 88*, 709-727.

Kohlberg, L. (1969). Stage and sequence: The cognitive developmental approach to socialization. In D.A. Goslin (Ed.), *Handbook of socialization theory and research.* Chicago: Rand McNally.

Kohlberg, L. (1971). From is to ought. In T. Mischel (Ed.), *Cognitive development and epistemology.* New York: Academic Press.

Kohlberg, L. (1976). Moral stages and moralization: The cognitive-developmental approach. In T. Lickona (Ed.), *Moral development and behavior.* New York: Holt, Rinehart, and Winston.

Kohlberg, L. (1984). *Essays on moral development Vol. II. The psychology of moral development.* San Fransisco: Harper & Row.

Kohlberg, L. & Candee, D. (1984). The relationship of moral judgment to moral action. In L. Kohlberg (Ed.), *Essays on moral development. Vol. II. The psychology of moral development* (pp. 498-620). San Fransisco: Harper and Row.

Kohlberg, L., Kauffman, K., Scharf, P. & Hickey, J. (1975). The just community approach to corrections: A theory. *Journal of Moral Education, 4*, 243-260.

Kohlberg, L. & Kramer, R. (1969). Continuities and discontinuities in childhood and adult moral development. *Human Development, 12*, 93-120.

Kohlberg, L., Levine, C. & Hewer, A. (1983). *Moral stages: A current formulation and a response to critics*. Basil: Karger.

Kuczynski, L. (1984). Socialization goals and mother-child interaction: Strategies for long-term and short-term compliance. *Developmental Psychology, 20*, 1061-1073.

Kuczynski, L., Kochanska, G., Radke-Yarrow, M. & Girnius-Brown, O. (1987). A developmental interpretation of young children's noncompliance. *Developmental Psychology, 23(6)*, 799-806.

Lepper, M. R. (1983). Social-control processes and the internalization of social values: an attributional perspective. In E.T. Higgins, D.N. Rubble, & W.W. Hartup (Eds.), *Social cognition and social development. A sociocultural perspective* (pp. 294-332). Cambridge: Cambridge University Press.

Lickona, T. (1980). Fostering moral development in the family. In D.B. Cochrane, & M. Manley-Casimir (Eds.), *Development of moral reasoning* (pp. 169-191). New York: Praeger.

Magmer, E. & Ipfling, H.J. (1973). Zum Problem des schichtenspezifischen Strafens. *Scienta Paedagogica Experimentalis, 10*, 170-192.

Matefy, R.E. & Acksen, B.A. (1976). The effect of role-playing discrepant positions on change in moral judgments and attitudes. *Journal of Genetic Psychology, 128*, 189-200.

Minton, C., Kagan, J. & Levine, J.A. (1971). Maternal control and obedience in the two-year-old. *Child Development, 42*, 1873-1894.

Mladek, G. (1982). Elterliches Reactionverhalten in fiktiven Eltern-Kind-Konfliktsituationen. *Acta Paedopsychiatrica, 48*, 27-32.

Mullhern, R.K. & Passman, R.H. (1981). Parental discipline as affected by the sex of the parent, the sex of the child, and the child's apparent responsiveness to discipline. *Developmental Psychology, 17*, 604-613.

Norcini, J.J. & Snyder, S.S. (1983). The effects of modeling and cognitive induction on the moral reasoning of adolescents. *Journal of Youth and Adolescence, 12*, 101-115.

Oldenshaw, L., Walters, G.C. & Hall, D.K. (1986). Control strategies and noncompliance in abusive mother-child dyads: An observational study. *Child Development, 57*, 722-732.

Olejnik, A.B. (1980). Adults' moral reasoning with children. *Child Development, 51*, 1285-1288.

Papini, D.R. (1987). Variations in conflictual family issues by adolescent pubertal status, gender, and family member. Paper presented at the Biennial Meeting of the Society for Research in Child Development. Baltimore MD.

Parikh, B. (1980). Development of moral judgment and its relation to family environmental factors in Indian and American families. *Child Development, 51* 1030-1039.

Patterson, G.R. (1980). Mothers: the unacknowledged victims. *Monographs of the Society for Research in Child Development, 45(5, Serial No. 186)*.

Patterson, G.R. (1982). *Coercive family process*. Eugene, OR: Castalia.

Perry, D.G., Perry, L.C. & Rasmussen, P. (1986). Cognitive social learning mediators of aggression. *Child Development, 57(3)*, 700-711.

Peterson, G.B., Hey, R.N. & Peterson, L.R. (1979). Intersection of family development and moral stage frameworks: Implications for theory and research. *Journal of the Marriage and the Family*, 229-235.

Peterson, C. & Skevington, S. (1987). The relation between young children's cognitive role-taking and mothers' preference for a conflict-inducing child rearing method. *Journal of Genetic Psychology, 149(2)*, 163-174.

Pettit, G.S. & Bayles, K.A. (1987). A taxonomy of family conflict situations. Paper presented at the Biennial Meeting of the Society for Research in Child Development. Baltimore MD.

Powers, S.I. (1988). Moral judgement development within the family. *Journal of Moral Education, 17(3)*, 209-219.

Radke-Yarrow, M., Zahn-Waxler, C. & Chapman, M. (1983). Children's prosocial dispositions and behavior. In P.H. Mussen (Ed.), *Handbook of child psychology. Vol. IV. Socialization, personality, and social development*. New York: Wiley.

Reid, B.V. & Valsinger, J. (1986). Consistency, praise, and love. Folk theories of American parents. *Ethos, 14*, 282-304.

Schnell, S. & Gibbs, J.C. (1987). Delinquents with mature moral reasoning: A comparison with delayed delinquents and mature nondelinquents. Paper presented at the Biennial Meeting of the Society for Research in Child Development. Baltimore MD.

Selman, R.L. (1976). Social-cognitive understanding. A guide to educational and clinical practice. In T. Lickona (Ed.), *Moral development and behavior*. New York: Holt, Rinehart, and Winston.

Selman, R.L. (1980). *The growth of interpersonal understanding: Developmental and clinical analyses*. New York: Academic Press.

Selman, R.L. & Byrne, D.F. (1974). A structural-developmental analysis of levels of role taking in middle childhood. *Child Development, 45*, 803-806.

Selman, R.L., Schorin, M.Z., Stone, C.R. & Phelps, E. (1983). A naturalistic study of children's social understanding. *Developmental Psychology, 19*, 82-102.

Shaffer, D.R. & Brody, G.H. (1981). Parental and peer influences on moral development. In R.W. Henderson (Ed.), *Parent-child interaction. Theory, research, and prospects*. New York: Academic Press.

Siebenheller, F.A. (1990). Problematische opvoedingssituaties: percepties, emoties en disciplineringsreacties van ouders. Dissertation, Catholic University of Nijmegen.

Simmons, H. & Schoggen, P. (1963). Mothers and fathers as sources of environmental pressure on children. In G. Barker (Ed.), *The stream of behavior*. (pp. 70-78). New York: Appleton-Century Crofts.

Slaby, R.G. & Guerra, N.G. (1988). Cognitive mediators of aggression in adolescent offenders: 1. Assessment. *Developmental Psychology, 24*, 580-588.

Smale, G.J.A. (1980). Psycho-sociale gevolgen en gedragsveranderingen bij slachtoffers van ernstige misdrijven. *Tijdschrift voor Criminologie, 22*, 223-241.

Smetana, J.G. (1984). Toddlers' social interactions regarding moral and conventional transgressions. *Child Development, 55*, 1767-1776.

Smetana, J.G. (1989). Toddlers' social interactions in the context of moral and conventional transgressions in the home. *Developmental Psychology, 25(4)*, 499-508.

Speicher, B. (1985a). Relationship between parent and offspring moral judgment: Longitudinal and cross-sectional age patterns. Paper presented at the Biennial Meeting of the Society for Research in Child Development. Toronto.

Speicher, B. (1985b). Family interaction and the development of moral judgment during adolescence. Paper presented at the Biennial Meeting of the Society for Research in Child Development. Toronto.

Stanley, S.F. (1978). Family education to enhance the moral atmosphere of the family and the moral development of adolescents. *Journal of Counseling Psychology, 25*, 110-118.

Stanley, S.F. (1980). The family and moral education. In R.L. Mosher (Ed.), *Moral Education*. (pp. 341-355). New York: Praeger.

Trevethan, S.D. & Walker, L.J. (1989). The moral development of psychopathic youths. Paper presented at the Biennial Meeting of the Society for Research in Child Development. Kansas City MO.

Trickett, P.K. & Kuczynski, L. (1986). Children's misbehaviors and parental discipline strategies in abusive and nonabusive families. *Developmental Psychology, 22*, 115-123.

Trickett, P.K. & Susman, E.J. (1988). Parental perceptions of child rearing practices in physically abusive and nonabusive families. *Developmental Psychology, 24(2)*, 270-276.

Vermulst, A.A., Gerris, J.R.M., Franken, W.M. & Janssens, J.M.A. (1986). Determinanten van ouderlijk functioneren tegen de achtergrond van de theorie van Kohn. In J.R.M. Gerris (Ed.), *Pedagogisch onderzoek in ontwikkeling* (pp. 19-42). Nijmegen: ITS.

Walker, L.J. (1982). The sequentiality of Kohlberg's stages of moral development. *Child Development, 53*, 1330-1336.

Walker, L.J. (1983). Sources of cognitive conflict for stage transition in moral development. *Developmental Psychology, 19*, 103-110.

Walker, L.J. (1989). Family patterns of moral reasoning. Paper presented at the Biennial Meeting of the Society for Research in Child Development. Kansas City MO.

Westerlaak, J.M. van, Kropman, J.A. & Collaris, J.W.M. (1975). *Beroepenklapper*. Nijmegen: ITS.

Wolfe, D.A., Fairbank, J.A., Kelly, J.A. & Bradlyn, A.S. (1983). Child abusive parents' physiological responses to stressful and non-stressful behavior in children. *Behavioral Assessment, 5*, 363-371.

Zahn-Waxler, C. & Chapman, M. (1982). Immediate antecedents of caretakers' methods of discipline. *Child Psychiatry and Human Development, 12*, 179-192.